The Unofficial Guide to Practical Skills

EDITION

2

The Unofficial Guide to Practical Skills

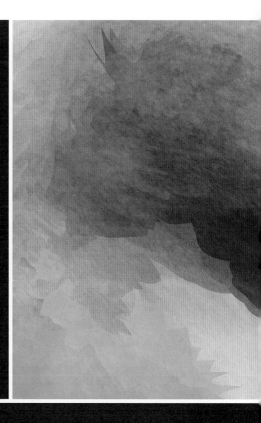

Series Editor

Zeshan Qureshi, BM, BSc (Hons), MSc, MRCPCH,
FAcadMEd, MRCPS(Glasg)
Paediatric Registrar
London Deanery
United Kingdom

Editors

Emily Hotton, MBChB (Dist), BSc (Hons) PhD, MRCOG
Women's and Children's Research
Southmead Hospital;
Translational Health Sciences
University of Bristol, Bristol
United Kingdom

Sammie Mak, MBChB
Junior Doctor
NHS England, Manchester
United Kingdom

ELSEVIER

Notices

Practitioners and researchers must always rely on their own experience and knowledge in evaluating and using any information, methods, compounds, or experiments described herein. Because of rapid advances in the medical sciences, in particular, independent verification of diagnoses and drug dosages should be made. To the fullest extent of the law, no responsibility is assumed by Elsevier, authors, editors, or contributors for any injury and/or damage to persons or property as a matter of products liability, negligence or otherwise, or from any use or operation of any methods, products, instructions, or ideas contained in the material herein.

ISBN: 978-0-323-93719-1

Content Strategist: Jeremy Bowes
Content Project Manager: Shubham Dixit
Design: Miles Hitchen
Illustration Manager: Akshaya Mohan
Marketing Manager: Deborah Watkins

Printed in India by Replika Press Pvt. Ltd.
Last digit is the print number: 9 8 7 6 5 4 3 2 1

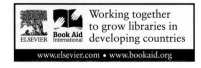

Series Editor Foreword

The Unofficial Guide to Medicine is not just about helping students study, it is also about allowing those that learn to take back control of their own education. Since its inception, it has been driven by the voices of students, and through this, democratised the process of medical education, blurring the line between learners and teachers.

Medical education is an evolving process, and the latest iteration of our titles has been rewritten to bring them up to date with modern curriculums, after extensive deliberation and consultation. We have kept the series up to date, incorporating new guidelines and perspectives from a wide range of students, junior doctors, and senior clinicians. There is greater consistency across the titles, more illustrations, and through these and other changes, I hope the books will now be even better study aids.

These books though are a process of continual improvement. By reading this book, I hope that you not only get through your exams but also consider contributing to a future edition. You may be a student now, but you are also the future of medical education.

I wish you all the best with your future career and any upcoming exams.

Zeshan Qureshi
November 2022

Introduction

The Unofficial Guide to Practical Skills is a crucial accompaniment to *The Unofficial Guide to Passing OSCEs*. This updated second edition covers the core clinical competencies for new graduates as outlined by the General Medical Council, as well as additional practical procedures that are expected to be performed by junior doctors and trainees. Written by recently qualified foundation doctors, with review by senior clinicians, we have ensured that all procedures follow current guidelines, wherever possible.

This book has detailed explanations of over 50 practical skills stations. Each station includes a corresponding mark scheme, associated questions and answers, as well as further areas to explore. The aim is to give you a comprehensive overview of all procedures, even if you have yet to witness them in your training. Covering both basic and more advanced practical skills, we hope this book will prove to be a handy study companion for your undergraduate and postgraduate training.

This book is useful for self-assessment, with informative fact boxes dispersed throughout to guide further learning. The included mark schemes will offer guidance for group study sessions with the opportunity to mark your colleagues.

Practical procedures can be nerve-wracking to perform, both under the close scrutiny of OSCE examiners and in the pressures of daily clinical practice. The following simple measures are central to performing practical skills proficiently and effectively:
- Take time to prepare yourself for the procedure.
- Ensure you are familiar with the method and equipment you need.
- Make sure that correct infection control measures are undertaken, from hand washing to use of personal protective items.
- Always identify the patient you are about to perform a procedure on and obtain the appropriate consent.
- Check that the patient understands your explanation and allow time for them to ask any questions.
- Be confident in your ability.
- Use the experience of your peers.
- If you are having difficulty, seek help.

With this textbook, we hope you will become more confident and competent in these skills, both in exams and in clinical practice, and we hope that this is just the beginning. We want you to get involved. This textbook has been written by junior doctors and students just like you because we believe:
- that fresh graduates have a unique perspective on what works *for students*. We have tried to capture the insight of students and recent graduates to make the language we use to discuss this complex material more digestible *for students*.
- that texts are in *constant* need of being updated. *Every student* has the potential to contribute to the education of others in innovative ways of thinking and learning. This book is an open collaboration with you.

You have the power to contribute something valuable to medicine; we welcome your suggestions and would love you to get in touch.

Emily Hotton, Sammie Mak and Zeshan Qureshi
November 2022

Acknowledgement

Thank you to below-listed contributors for their contribution to 1st edition:

Natalie Blencowe
Associate Professor in Surgery
Bristol Medical School (PHS)
University of Bristol, England

Andiran Anduvan
Core Medical Trainee
Charles University, Prague

Srikant Ganesh
Foundation Doctor
University of Bristol, England

Nikki Hall
Opthalmology Trainee
University of Edinburgh, Scotland

Ruth Harrison
Foundation Doctor
University of Bristol, England

James Hayward
Foundation Doctor
University of Bristol, England

Katrina Mason
Core Surgical Trainee
University of Bristol, England

Abbreviations and Symbols

°	degrees
ABPI	ankle brachial pressure index
AMD	age-related macular degeneration
β	beta
BE	base excess
BiPAP	bilevel positive airway pressure
BMI	body mass index
BP	blood pressure
cm	centimetre(s)
cmH_2O	centimetre of water
CO_2	carbon dioxide
COPD	chronic obstructive pulmonary disease
CPAP	continuous positive airway pressure
CPR	cardiopulmonary resuscitation
CRP	C reactive protein
CSF	cerebrospinal fluid
CT	computed tomography
CVP	central venous pressure
DKA	diabetic ketoacidosis
DLCO	diffusion capacity of the lung for carbon monoxide
ECG	electrocardiogram
EDTA	ethylenediaminetetraacetic acid
FBC	full blood count
FEV_1	forced expiratory volume in one second
FiO_2	inspired oxygen concentration
FVC	forced vital capacity
GCS	Glasgow Coma Score
Hb	haemoglobin
HCO_3^-	bicarbonate
HAS	human albumin solution
ICP	intracranial pressure
ID	identification
IJV	internal jugular vein
INR	international normalised ratio
IV	intravenous
kg	kilograms
kPa	kilopascal(s) pressure
L	litre
LA	local anaesthetic
LFTs	liver function tests
LP	lumbar puncture
m	metres
MC&S	microscopy, culture and sensitivity
mg	milligram(s)
MI	myocardial infarction
min	minute(s)
mL	millilitre(s)
mmHg	millimetres of mercury pressure
mmol	millimoles
MRSA	methicillin-resistant Staphylococcus aureus
NPDR	non-proliferative diabetic retinopathy
NTT	non-touch technique
O_2	oxygen
OP	oropharyngeal
$PaCO_2$	arterial partial pressure of carbon dioxide
PaO_2	arterial partial pressure of oxygen
PCI	primary coronary intervention
PEA	pulseless electrical activity
PICC	peripherally inserted central catheter
PPE	personal protective equipment
PT	prothrombin time
SaO_2	arterial oxygen saturation
SAAG	serum-ascites albumin gradient
SBP	spontaneous bacterial peritonitis
STEMI	ST elevation myocardial infarction
TB	tuberculosis
TLCO	transfer factor of the lung for carbon monoxide
U&E	urea and electrolyte
USS	ultrasound scan
VF	ventricular fibrillation
VT	ventricular tachycardia
WCC	white cell count

Contents

Basic Patient Assessment

Outline

STATION 1.1: HEART RATE AND RESPIRATORY RATE

SCENARIO

You are a junior doctor working in the emergency department (ED) and have been asked to see Mrs Bradbury, a 60-year-old woman, who has presented with pelvic pain. Please accurately measure and record her heart rate and respiratory rate.

OBJECTIVES

- Accurately measure and interpret the heart rate
- Accurately measure and interpret the respiratory rate
- Accurately record the heart rate and respiratory rate on a National Early Warning Score (NEWS) chart

GENERAL ADVICE

1. Always wash your hands before and after patient contact.
2. Obtain consent before starting the procedure.
3. At the end of the procedure, discuss your findings with the patient and record them appropriately in the notes.
4. Thank the patient for her time, and ensure that she is comfortable.
5. Give her privacy to get dressed again if required.

MEASURING HEART RATE

- Check that the patient is in a comfortable position with the arm supported and the lower arm exposed.
- Place your index and middle finger pads over the lateral aspect of the wrist at the site of the radial pulse (Fig. 1.1).
- Once identified, assess the rate and rhythm of the radial pulse for 1 min (in practice, this is usually assessed over 15 s and multiplied by 4).
- Document your findings in the patient's notes.
- Rate: Recorded as beats/min (bpm). See Table 1.1.
- Rhythm: See Table 1.2.

MEASURING RESPIRATORY RATE

- Check that the patient is in a comfortable position with the chest exposed.
- Watch the chest for movement. If this is subtle, explain to the patient that you are going to place your hand on her chest to feel for chest wall movement.
- Assess the respiratory rate and regularity for 1 min (Table 1.3).
- Document your findings in the patient's notes.

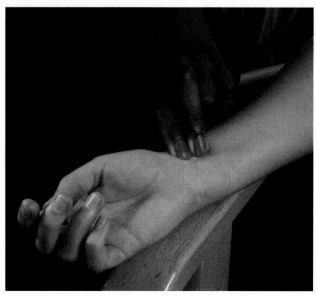

Fig. 1.1 Palpate the radial pulse with the pads of your fingers.

Table 1.1   Interpreting Heart Rate

RATE DESCRIPTION	BPM
Tachycardia	>100
Bradycardia	<60

Table 1.2   Causes of Different Heart Rhythms

RHYTHM	CAUSES
Regular	• Sinus rhythm
Regularly irregular	• Sinus arrhythmia • Second-degree heart block
Irregularly irregular	• Atrial or ventricular ectopics • Atrial fibrillation (some cases of atrial flutter with variable heart block)

Table 1.3   Respiratory Rate Changes With Age

AGE	NORMAL (BREATHS/MIN)	TACHYPNOEA (BREATHS/MIN)
Neonate	30–50	>60
5–12 months	30–40	>50
1–5 years	25–30	>40
5–12 years	20–25	>30
>12 years	12–20	>20

Present Your Findings

Today I measured the heart rate and respiratory rate of Mrs Bradbury, a 60-year-old woman. Her pulse rate was regular at 84 bpm and of good volume, whereas her respiratory rate was 16 breaths/min. Both of these were within normal limits. I would also like to measure the other vital signs in order to calculate a NEWS.

QUESTIONS AND ANSWERS FOR CANDIDATE

Name three medications that can cause tachycardia.
• Levothyroxine
• Salbutamol
• Duloxetine
• Venlafaxine
• Amitriptyline

Name three medications that can cause bradycardia.
• Propranolol
• Digoxin
• Amlodipine
• Diltiazem
• Propofol

What are the commonest physiological causes of bradycardia?
• Being an athlete
• Sleep

Mark Scheme for Examiner

	0	1	2	3
Introduction and General Preparation				
Introduces self and washes hands				
Confirms patient's identity with three points of identification				
Explains procedure, identifies concerns and obtains consent				
Measuring the Heart Rate				
Exposes the wrist and supports the arm; ensures patient is comfortable				
Correctly identifies anatomical location				
Assesses heart rate for 1 min				
Measuring the Respiratory Rate				
Ensures adequate view of patient's chest; ensures patient is comfortable				
Assesses respiratory rate for 1 min				
Finishing				
Documents findings on NEWS chart and in patient's notes				
Thanks the patient for his/her time, and gives the patient privacy to get dressed again if required				
Discusses findings with the patient				

0 = Not attempted
1 = Performed, with room for improvement
2 = Adequately performed
3 = Performed beyond level expected

Name two pathological causes of bradycardia.
- Pharmacological: Any negative chronotrope; for example, beta-blockers
- Acute myocardial infarction (MI): Particularly an inferior MI leading to a heart block
- Cushing's reflex: A systemic reaction to raised intracranial pressure, including bradycardia, erratic breathing and widened pulse pressure
- Hypoxia
- Hypothermia
- Hypothyroidism

Name three causes of tachypnoea.
- Physiological: Exercise, anxiety, excitement
- Circulatory shock: Septic shock, anaphylactic shock, hypovolaemic shock
- Lung pathology: Pneumonia, asthma, pneumothorax
- Other pathology: Heart failure, anaemia, myocardial infarction

 Tip Box

It is best to count the respiratory rate when the patient is unaware—for example, when you are taking the pulse rate—otherwise it can unknowingly increase the patient's anxiety and therefore the respiratory rate.

 Fact Box

If there is a delay between the bilateral radial pulses, known as radio-radial delay, this suggests a narrowing of the aorta which could be attributed to aortic coarctation, subclavian stenosis and Takayasu arteritis.

STATION 1.2: OXYGEN SATURATION

SCENARIO

You are a junior doctor on the ward and Mr Michael, an 80-year-old non-binary person, has just walked back from the toilet and now feels breathless. Please record his oxygen saturation.

OBJECTIVE

- Measuring and interpreting oxygen saturation

GENERAL ADVICE

- Always wash your hands before and after patient contact and obtain consent before starting the procedure.
- At the end of the procedure, discuss your findings with the patient and record them appropriately in the notes. Remember pulse oximeters may be less reliable in those with increased skin pigmentation.

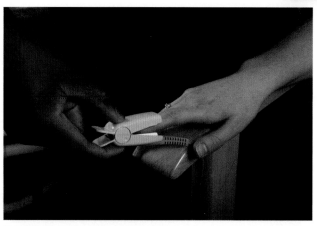

Fig. 1.2 Ensure that the probe is placed on the finger with the sensor on the dorsal aspect of the hand.

EQUIPMENT

- Oxygen saturation probe

MEASURING OXYGEN SATURATION

1. Ensure that the patient is comfortable and elect a forefinger that is clean and without nail polish (Fig. 1.2).
2. Correctly position the oxygen saturation probe onto the end of the forefinger, and ensure the machine is turned on.
3. Read off the oxygen saturation.
4. Note whether the patient is breathing room air or is receiving supplementary oxygen.

 Present Your Findings

Today I measured the oxygen saturation of Mr Michael, an 80-year-old man. His oxygen saturation measured 96%, which is within normal limits. I would also like to measure the other vital signs in order to calculate a NEWS.

? QUESTIONS AND ANSWERS FOR CANDIDATE

Where can an oxygen probe be placed?
- Finger
- Toe
- Ear lobe

Name two causes of hypoxaemia.
- Low concentration of inspired oxygen; for example, breathing at high altitude
- Right-to-left shunting (blood bypasses the lungs); for example, Eisenmenger's syndrome
- Ventilation—perfusion mismatch; for example, pneumonia, pulmonary oedema
- Diffusion impairment; for example, interstitial lung disease

Mark Scheme for Examiner

	0	1	2	3
Introduction and General Preparation				
Introduces self and washes hands				
Confirms patient's identity with three points of identification				
Explains procedure, identifies concerns and obtains consent				
Measuring Oxygen Saturation				
Exposes the patient's hand and ensures no nail polish (if applicable)				
Checks if the patient is on supplementary oxygen				
Positions probe correctly onto finger				
Finishing				
Documents findings on NEWS chart and in patient's notes				
Thanks the patient for his time, and gives the patient privacy to get dressed again if required				
Discusses findings with the patient				

0 = Not attempted
1 = Performed, with room for improvement
2 = Adequately performed
3 = Performed beyond level expected

- Hypoventilation; for example, brainstem tumour, intracerebral haemorrhage, Guillain–Barré syndrome

What are the different ways you might deliver oxygen?
- Nasal cannula
- Simple face mask
- Venturi mask
- Non-rebreathe mask
- Tracheostomy mask

What is the normal range of oxygen saturations?
- A patient's oxygen saturation in a healthy adult should be 94%–98% without any supplementary oxygen.

What are the different concentrations that a Venturi mask can come in?
- 24%
- 28%
- 31%
- 35%
- 40%
- 60%

 Tip Box

If a patient is wearing nail polish, try to remove this before taking an oxygen saturation reading.

 Fact Box

Cerebral anoxia refers to a complete interruption of the supply of oxygen to the brain, whereas cerebral hypoxia refers to a partial interruption of the supply of oxygen to the brain.

STATION 1.3: BLOOD PRESSURE

SCENARIO

You are a junior doctor on the ward and Mrs Space, a 50-year-old woman, has recently stopped her anti-hypertensive medication. Please check her blood pressure (BP).

OBJECTIVE

- Measuring and interpreting BP using manual and electronic techniques

GENERAL ADVICE

1. Always wash your hands before and after patient contact and obtain consent before performing the procedure.
2. Ensure that the patient is comfortable and adequately expose the right arm.
3. Correctly position the arm so it is supported. The point at which you will measure the BP in the arm should be approximately level with the heart.
4. Select an appropriately sized cuff.
5. At the end of the procedure discuss your findings with the patient and record them appropriately in the notes.

EQUIPMENT

- BP machine
- BP cuff

MEASURING BLOOD PRESSURE

FOR THE MANUAL TECHNIQUE

1. Correctly place the BP cuff on the patient's arm (Fig. 1.3).
2. Locate the brachial artery (usually found at the medial border of the antecubital fossa, medial to the biceps tendon).
3. Inflate the cuff until the pulse becomes impalpable.
4. Note the pressure on the manometer.
5. Deflate the cuff and place the stethoscope over the brachial artery (Fig. 1.4).
6. Reinflate the cuff to a pressure 20 mmHg higher than that noted previously.
7. Deflate the cuff by 2 mmHg/s at a time.
8. Note the pressure at which you hear the first heart sounds (systolic BP).
9. Continue to deflate the cuff and note the pressure at which heart sounds completely disappear (diastolic BP).

FOR AN AUTOMATIC ELECTRONIC DEVICE

1. Correctly place the BP cuff on the patient's arm (Fig. 1.3).
2. Switch on the BP device and press the start button.

3. Note the BP reading and document your findings on the patient's observation chart.

Present Your Findings

Today I measured the blood pressure of Mrs Space, a 50-year-old woman, after her recent anti-hypertensive medication was stopped. Her blood pressure today was 131/87 mmHg. This is within her target blood pressure range. I would also like to measure the other vital signs in order to calculate a NEWS and ask her primary care physician to recheck her home blood pressure in 1–2 weeks' time.

? QUESTIONS AND ANSWERS FOR CANDIDATE

What can make a BP recording inaccurate?
- If the patient is anxious
- If the patient has not adequately rested before the BP reading
- If the BP cuff size is incorrect
- If only one BP reading is taken

In what situations would it be advisable to take the BP from the left arm?

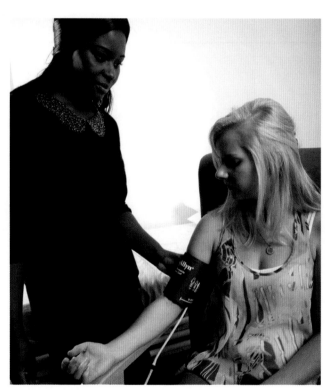

Fig. 1.3 The patient's arm should be positioned so that it is at the level of the heart.

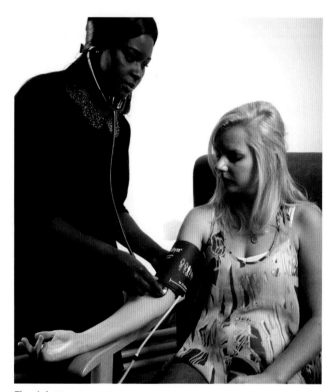

Fig. 1.4 Use the stethoscope to determine the systolic and diastolic pressures.

Mark Scheme for Examiner

	0	1	2	3
Introduction and General Preparation				
Introduces self and washes hands				
Confirms patient's identity with three points of identification				
Explains procedure, identifies concerns and obtains consent				
Exposes right arm (or left arm if any issues with using right arm)				
Positions arm BP measurement point at the level of the heart				
Selects and applies an appropriately sized cuff				
Measuring the Blood Pressure — Manual Technique				
Palpates the brachial artery				
Inflates the cuff to systole				
Deflates the cuff				
Positions the stethoscope				
Reinflates the cuff to 20 mmHg above systole				
Deflates the cuff at the appropriate rate				
Notes the systolic and diastolic pressures				
Measuring the Blood Pressure — Automatic Electronic Device				
Switches on the machine and starts the recording				
Reads the BP correctly				
Finishing				
Documents findings on NEWS chart and in patient's notes				
Thanks the patient for her time, and gives the patient privacy to get dressed again if required				
Discusses findings with the patient				

0 = Not attempted
1 = Performed, with room for improvement
2 = Adequately performed
3 = Performed beyond level expected

- If the right arm has an intravenous (IV) infusion in situ
- If the right arm is paralysed
- If there is lymphoedema in the right arm
- If there is a fistula in the right arm
- Patient preference

What is malignant hypertension, and how do you manage it?
- Malignant hypertension is a specific form of hypertension that is a medical emergency, as diastolic BP may rise to >130 mmHg.
- If the patient has severe hypertension (clinic BP>180/120 mmHg) but no signs or symptoms indicating same-day referral, then carry out investigations for target organ damage as soon as possible.
- If the patient has severe hypertension (clinic BP>180/120 mmHg) as well as any of the following signs or symptoms, then refer the patient for same-day specialist assessment:
  - Signs of retinal haemorrhage or papilloedema
  - New-onset confusion
  - Chest pain
  - Signs of heart failure
  - Acute kidney injury
  - Suspected phaeochromocytoma

What lifestyle advice can be given to patients with hypertension?
- Reduce salt intake
- Eat a well-balanced diet
- Increase the level of physical activity
- Avoid smoking
- Avoid alcohol consumption
- Reduce and manage mental stress

What are the common first-line medications for hypertension?
- For someone <55 years old *and* not from an Afro-Caribbean or Black-African ethnicity, offer an angiotensin-converting enzyme inhibitor (ACEi) or angiotensin II receptor blocker (ARB).
- For someone >55 years old *or* any age but from an Afro-Caribbean or Black-African ethnicity, offer a calcium channel blocker. Note that ethnicity-based prescribing for hypertension whilst recommended in 2019 NICE guidance is controversial and not universally agreed upon.

 Tip Box

Ensure that the patient does not talk whilst you are taking the BP. If the patient is talking it may change the reading, and silence will help you to hear better.

Fact Box

The systolic BP represents the pressure in the blood vessels when the heart contracts. Diastolic BP represents the pressure in the blood vessels when the heart relaxes.

STATION 1.4: LYING AND STANDING BLOOD PRESSURE

SCENARIO

You are a junior doctor on the ward and Mrs Monty, a 69-year-old woman, presents to you in the ED with recurrent falls. Please perform a lying and standing BP and relay your findings.

OBJECTIVES

- Performing lying and standing BP
- Interpreting the results of lying and standing BP

GENERAL ADVICE

- Lying and standing BP can be used to diagnose (or demonstrate) postural hypotension. Ensure that you have the time to perform the examination properly and you are not rushing the patient, as this may falsely elevate the BP reading.

EQUIPMENT

- BP machine
- BP cuff

MEASURING LYING AND STANDING BLOOD PRESSURE

1. Introduce yourself to the patient and obtain consent.
2. Position the patient supine and ensure that she has been lying there for at least 5 min (Fig. 1.5).
3. Take the patient's BP as outlined in station 1.3.
4. Document the lying systolic and diastolic pressures.
5. Leave the cuff in place and ask the patient to stand (Fig. 1.6).
6. Inform the patient that she needs to stand for 1 min before you will retake the BP.
7. Ensure the arm is supported at the level of the heart.
8. Retake the BP as outlined previously.
9. Remove the cuff and allow the patient to sit.
10. Document the standing systolic and diastolic pressures.
11. Explain your findings to the patient.

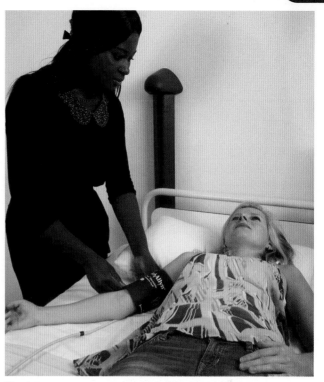

Fig. 1.5 Ensure correct positioning of patient and BP cuff.

DOCUMENTING THE LYING AND STANDING BLOOD PRESSURE

1. Document the patient's BP after the patient has been lying down for at least 5 min.
2. Document the patient's BP after the patient has been standing up for at least 1 min.
3. Work out the difference between the lying BP and standing BP, and document whether this is positive or negative for postural hypotension.

Present Your Findings

Mrs Monty is a 69-year-old woman who has presented with a fall. On examination, her lying BP was 146/82 mmHg and her standing BP was 118/79 mmHg. She therefore has a postural systolic drop of greater than 20 mmHg, which is suggestive of postural hypo-tension. I would like to determine the cause of her postural hypotension, so I would take a full history and examine her with a particular focus on the cardiovascular exam and her fluid status. I would also look at the observation chart and review her current medications.

❓ QUESTIONS AND ANSWERS FOR CANDIDATE

How would you define postural hypotension?

- Postural (or orthostatic) hypotension is defined as a fall in systolic BP >20 mmHg or a drop in diastolic BP >10 mmHg when a patient assumes a standing position as compared to when lying down.

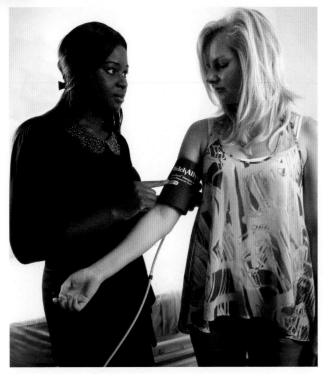

Fig. 1.6 The BP cuff can be kept in situ between lying and standing.

Describe the management for a well patient with postural hypotension.
- Treat any reversible cause; for example, poor fluid intake or medications like antihypertensives.
- Use conservative measures; for example, the patient should not stand up too quickly.
- Compression bandaging could be considered to improve venous return.
- If conservative measures fail, consider specific medication; for example, fludrocortisone.

What are the symptoms of postural hypotension?
- Asymptomatic
- Dizziness
- Lightheadedness
- Temporary loss of consciousness
- Symptoms that occur on standing

What is a tilt table test?
- The patient lies flat on a specially designed table or bed while connected to an electrocardiogram (ECG) and BP monitors. This bed can be tilted from the lying to standing position, and when this is performed, autonomic reflex testing will allow clinicians to determine whether the cause of the postural hypotension is neurogenic or not.

Mark Scheme for Examiner

	0	1	2	3
Introduction and General Preparation				
Introduces self and washes hands				
Confirms patient's identity with three points of identification				
Explains procedure, identifies concerns and obtains consent				
Measuring the Lying Blood Pressure				
Positions the patient supine				
Leaves the patient lying for at least 5 min				
Takes the lying BP and documents it				
Measuring the Standing Blood Pressure				
Leaves the cuff in place				
Asks the patient to stand				
Leaves the patient standing for 1 min				
Retakes the standing BP and documents it				
Finishing				
Removes the cuff and allows the patient to sit				
Documents the findings in the patient's notes				
Thanks the patient for her time, and gives her privacy to get dressed again if required				
Discusses findings with the patient				

0 = Not attempted
1 = Performed, with room for improvement
2 = Adequately performed
3 = Performed beyond level expected

What is postural orthostatic tachycardia syndrome?
- It is an abnormal increase in heart rate that occurs after sitting or standing up. This is due to a flaw in the autonomic nervous system. There is a reduction in blood supply to the heart and brain upon becoming upright, therefore the heart rate increases to compensate.

 Tip Box

Some patients are unable to tolerate lying flat for long periods of time. Before you ask them to lie flat, ensure that you ask them if they are able to lie flat. If they are unable to lie completely flat, be aware that your examination findings may need to be interpreted with caution. Alternatively, you may wish to pragmatically do a sitting BP instead of a lying BP.

 Fact Box

The most common medications that may contribute to orthostatic hypotension include: beta-blockers, diuretics, ACEi, phenothiazines, ʟ-dopa and tranquillisers.

STATION 1.5: ANKLE BRACHIAL PRESSURE INDEX

SCENARIO

Mr Fisher is a 68-year-old man who presents to your clinic with pain and cramping in his left lower leg. The pain occurs on walking and is relieved by rest. Mr Fisher is a smoker and is receiving medical treatment for hyperlipidaemia and hypertension. Please measure the ankle brachial pressure index (ABPI) and tell the examiner your interpretation of the findings.

OBJECTIVE

- Measuring and interpreting ABPI readings

GENERAL ADVICE

- Make sure that you have protected any ulcers that may be present.

EQUIPMENT

- BP machine
- BP cuff
- Doppler gel
- Doppler probe

MEASURING ABPI

1. Introduce yourself to the patient and obtain consent.

2. Position the patient supine to remove the effect of gravity on blood flow.
3. Place an appropriately sized cuff around the right calf.
4. Locate the dorsalis pedis or posterior tibial pulse (Fig. 1.7).
5. Place the Doppler gel and probe on the skin near to where you expect to find the pulse (Fig. 1.8).
6. Listen for the sound of blood flow, a 'whoosh-whoosh' sound.
7. Inflate the cuff until the sound of blood flow has disappeared.
8. Deflate the cuff by 2 mmHg/s until you hear the blood flow returning and note this ankle systolic pressure.
9. Place an appropriately sized cuff around the patient's right arm.
10. Locate the brachial pulse at the medial border of the antecubital fossa (Fig. 1.9).
11. Repeat steps 5–8, noting the brachial systolic pressure.
12. Repeat steps 3–11 in the opposite limbs.

13. Calculate the **ABPI** $= \dfrac{\text{Ankle Systolic Pressure}}{\text{Brachial Systolic Pressure}}$

14. Explain the significance of ABPI to the patient, and document your findings.

Interpretation of ABPI

ABPI <0.5	ABPI 0.5–0.8	ABPI 0.9–1.2	ABPI >1.3
Severe arterial disease	Moderate arterial disease	Within the normal range	May indicate calcified arteries (and may mask underlying stenosis)

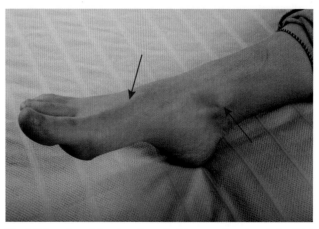

Fig. 1.7 Location of the dorsalis pedis (blue arrow) and posterior tibial (red arrow) pulses.

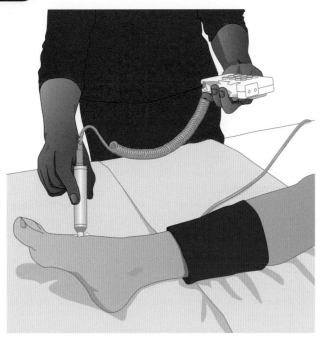

Fig. 1.8 Carefully locate the best position to listen to the sound of blood flow with the Doppler.

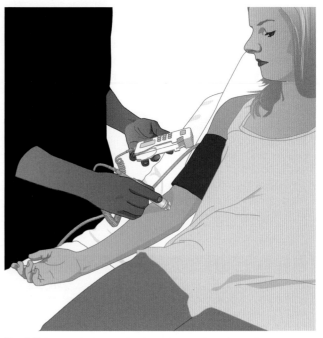

Fig. 1.9 Locate the brachial pulse using the Doppler probe.

Mark Scheme for Examiner

	0	1	2	3
Introduction and General Preparation				
Introduces self and washes hands				
Confirms patient's identity with three points of identification				
Explains procedure, identifies concerns and obtains consent				
Positions patient supine				
Measuring Ankle Systolic Pressure				
Selects and applies an appropriately sized cuff to the calf				
Palpates a peripheral pulse				
Places the Doppler gel and probe over the artery				
Inflates the cuff to above systole				
Deflates the cuff				
Records the systolic pressure				
Measuring the Brachial Systolic Pressure				
Selects and applies an appropriately sized cuff to arm				
Palpates the brachial pulse				
Places the Doppler gel and probe over the artery				
Inflates the cuff to above systole				
Deflates the cuff				
Records the systolic pressure				
Repeats on the opposite limb				
Calculating the ABPI				
Correctly calculates the ABPI				

Mark Scheme for Examiner—cont'd

	0	1	2	3
Finishing				
Wipes any Doppler gel from the patient				
Documents findings in patient's notes				
Thanks the patient for his time, and gives the patient privacy to get dressed again if required				
Discusses findings with the patient				

0 = Not attempted
1 = Performed, with room for improvement
2 = Adequately performed
3 = Performed beyond level expected

Present Your Findings

Mr Fisher is a 68-year-old man who has presented with intermittent claudication. He has known hypertension and hyperlipidaemia. On examination, his ankle systolic pressure is 80 mmHg and his brachial systolic pressure is 130 mmHg. His ABPI is therefore 0.6; this result, in conjunction with his symptoms, suggests peripheral vascular disease. I would like to take a full history, and examination. He may benefit from referral to the vascular surgeons and imaging, such as an arterial duplex scan.

QUESTIONS AND ANSWERS FOR CANDIDATE

How might you investigate someone with an ABPI suggesting peripheral vascular disease?
- I would check the patient's blood sugar and lipid profile because of possible underlying atherosclerosis. An ECG may also be helpful if there are any concerns about associated ischaemic heart disease. I would then refer the patient for an arterial duplex scan. The patient may also benefit from computed tomography or magnetic resonance angiogram.

Name four risk factors for peripheral arterial disease.
- Smoking
- Obesity
- Hypertension
- Hypercholesterolaemia
- Diabetes
- Male
- Family history

Name three symptoms of peripheral arterial disease.
- Pain in legs when walking, which may disappear after a period of rest
- Hair loss on legs and feet
- Paraesthesia in the legs
- Leg weakness
- Lower-limb ulcers
- Lower-limb skin discoloration

What are the signs of acute limb ischaemia?
- Pain
- Pallor
- Paralysis
- Pulselessness
- Paraesthesia
- Poikilothermia
- Gangrene
- Shiny, smooth lower limbs

What is the anatomical location of the dorsalis pedis pulse?
- On the dorsum of the foot, deep to the inferior extensor retinaculum and lying between the extensor hallucis longus tendon and medial tendon of the extensor digitorum longus muscle

Tip Box

ABPI should always be undertaken before applying a compression bandage to ensure there is no underlying arterial disease.

Fact Box

Patients with diabetes often have blood vessels that are calcified, which are less compressible and therefore may give a misleadingly high ABPI result.

STATION 1.6: BLOOD GLUCOSE

SCENARIO

Mrs Juniper, a 27-year-old woman, is a type 1 diabetic, on insulin. Please record Mrs Juniper's blood glucose before her lunch.

OBJECTIVE

- Measuring and interpreting blood glucose

GENERAL ADVICE

1. Obtain consent.
2. Ensure you wear gloves for this procedure.
3. Before approaching the patient, check that the blood glucose monitor is working and has been calibrated correctly, and that the recording strips are in date.

4. At the end of the procedure, discuss your findings with the patient and record them appropriately in the notes.

EQUIPMENT CHECKLIST

(Remember to check expiry dates on all equipment.)
- Tray: Either single-use, disposable sterilised tray or a decontaminated plastic tray that is cleaned pre/post-procedure
- Single-use disposable apron
- Non-sterile glove
- Skin-cleansing solution
- Cotton wool
- Glucose test strips
- Glucometer
- Blood lancet
- Plaster
- Sharps bin: The sharps bin should always be taken to the point of care.

Note: Skin-cleansing solutions and method will vary depending on local policy. If taking blood cultures, blood culture bottle ports will need to be fully cleaned and allowed to dry fully before use.

MEASURING BLOOD GLUCOSE

1. Establish when the patient last ate.
2. Ensure the patient is comfortable and clean the target finger with cotton wool and water or skin-cleansing solution.
3. Put on a pair of non-sterile gloves.
4. Insert a test strip into the glucose monitor.

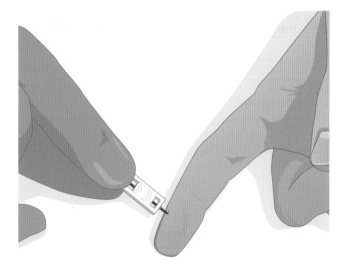

Fig. 1.10 Always use the side of the finger.

5. On the side of the finger, use a single-use lancet to prick the finger and immediately dispose of the lancet in a sharps bin (Fig. 1.10).
6. Wait for a drop of blood to appear.
7. Slowly bring the tip of the test strip perpendicular to the blood drop. As the strip touches the blood, a small amount of blood should be absorbed into the electronic part of the test strip. A beep signifies this has happened correctly (Fig. 1.11).
8. Wait for the result to be calculated.
9. Stop any bleeding with cotton wool and apply a plaster if necessary.

🔍 Mark Scheme for Examiner

	0	1	2	3
Introduction and General Preparation				
Introduces self and washes hands				
Confirms patient's identity with three points of identification				
Explains procedure, identifies concerns and obtains consent				
Checks the blood glucose machine and recording strips				
Checks the test finger is clean				
Checks when the patient last ate				
Measuring Blood Glucose				
Inserts a recording strip into the machine				
Dons non-sterile gloves				
Pricks finger with lancet				
Applies blood to the recording strip				
Waits for the result to be calculated				
Finishing				
Stops any bleeding with cotton wool				
Disposes of the recording strip				
Removes gloves and washes hands				

Mark Scheme for Examiner—cont'd

	0	1	2	3
Documents findings in patient's notes				
Thanks the patient for her time, and gives the patient privacy to get dressed again if required				
Discusses findings with the patient				

0 = Not attempted
1 = Performed, with room for improvement
2 = Adequately performed
3 = Performed beyond level expected

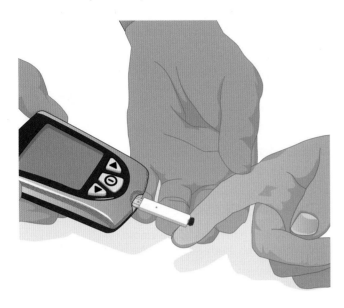

Fig. 1.11 Make sure you have enough blood to coat the end of the test strip fully.

10. Dispose of the test strip and wash your hands.
11. Document your findings in the patient's notes.

Present Your Findings

Today I took the blood glucose level of Mrs Juniper, a 27-year-old type 1 diabetic, on insulin, before her lunch. It measured 7.0 mmol/L, which is within range and expected for a diabetic patient who has been fasting. I have emphasised to Mrs Juniper the importance of checking her blood glucose level at least four times a day to reduce her risk of hypoglycaemia.

? QUESTIONS AND ANSWERS FOR CANDIDATE

How might you measure long-term blood glucose control in a diabetic?
- HbA1c test, which indicates the blood glucose control over the previous 3 months

Give two risk factors for type 2 diabetes.
- Hypertension
- Hypercholesterolaemia
- Previous gestational diabetes
- Increased body mass index (BMI)
- Family history of type 2 diabetes
- Older age

Give three complications of diabetes.
- Diabetic nephropathy
- Diabetic retinopathy
- Diabetic neuropathy
- Diabetic foot ulcers
- Macrovascular disease; for example, myocardial infarction and stroke

How might a hypoglycaemic episode present?
- Confusion or drowsiness
- Hunger
- Sweatiness
- Tingling lips
- Tremors
- Dizziness
- Seizures

How do you manage hypoglycaemia in someone with type 1 diabetes, on insulin?
- Any insulin infusions should be ceased.
- Patients with a blood glucose concentration >4 mmol/L but with hypoglycaemic symptoms should be given a small carbohydrate snack; for example, a slice of bread.
- Patients with a blood glucose concentration <4 mmol/L with or without symptoms, and who are conscious and can swallow, should have 15–20 g fast-acting carbohydrate; for example, glucose tablets. This can be repeated after 10–15 min up to a total of three treatments.
- If the blood glucose concentration is still <4 mmol/L then the patient should be treated with intramuscular glucagon or 10% glucose intravenously.
- A long-acting carbohydrate should be given once the patient has recovered and blood glucose concentration >4 mmol/L.

Tip Box

If you are struggling to obtain enough blood, move the patient's hand downward to let gravity assist. You can also 'milk' the finger by squeezing blood distally towards the fingerprick site.

Fact Box

The reason that 50% glucose infusion is not recommended is because it is hypertonic and would therefore increase the risk of extravasation injury. It is always viscous, which would make administration difficult.

STATION 1.7: MRSA SWAB

SCENARIO

Mr Nut, a 20-year-old man, is attending a preoperative appointment. Please perform a methicillin-resistant *Staphylococcus aureus* (MRSA) swab on him.

OBJECTIVE

- Performing an MRSA swab

GENERAL ADVICE

- Ensure you wear gloves for this procedure and obtain consent.
- Explain to the patient why hospital policy requires every patient to have an MRSA swab on admission – determining whether a patient has MRSA before admission allows prompt treatment to remove the bacteria.

EQUIPMENT

- Non-sterile gloves
- Nasal swab

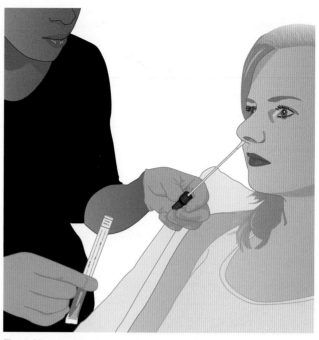

Fig. 1.12 Swab the inside of the nose gently.

PERFORMING AN MRSA SWAB

1. Ensure the patient is comfortable.
2. Gently swab both sides of the nasal septum and through both nostrils with a single swab (Fig. 1.12).
   Note: Swabs should not be moistened; the only exception is for very dry skin sites. For these, swabs moistened with sterile water can be used.
3. Place swabs in transport medium and specify MRSA screening on the request form.
4. Document in the notes that MRSA screening has been performed and that the results are pending.

Mark Scheme for Examiner

	0	1	2	3
Introduction and General Preparation				
Introduces self and washes hands				
Confirms patient's identity with three points of identification				
Explains procedure, identifies concerns and obtains consent				
Performing an MRSA Swab				
Washes hands and dons non-sterile gloves				
Swabs both nostrils with a single swab				
Places swab in transport medium				
Finishing				
Correctly labels the swab and request form				
Removes gloves and washes hands				
Thanks the patient for his time				
Informs the patient when the results are likely to be ready				

0 = Not attempted
1 = Performed, with room for improvement
2 = Adequately performed
3 = Performed beyond level expected

QUESTIONS AND ANSWERS FOR CANDIDATE

What happens if an inpatient is found to be MRSA-positive?
- The patient will be moved to a side room and barrier-nursed.
- The patient will be started on treatment according to the hospital policy.
- In the context of a suspected infection in the patient, your antimicrobial options would have to consider covering MRSA infection.

How is MRSA spread?
- It is primarily spread by physical contact. This is either direct skin-to-skin contact or contact with an object contaminated with MRSA.

How can the spread of MRSA be prevented?
- Maintain good hand hygiene and regular hand washing.
- Clean surfaces regularly.
- Use of personal protective equipment (PPE) appropriately.
- Reduce moments of direct contact.
- Avoid sharing objects, especially personal items such as towels, clothes and bedding.

Name two other infections that require patients to be in side rooms.
- Gastroenteritis
- Head lice
- Meningitis

Which patients are more vulnerable to contracting MRSA infections?
- Immunocompromised individuals
- Patients with open wounds

 Tip Box

Practise snapping off the swab at the breakline because it is not easy to tell if it's your first time doing it!

 Fact Box

If the patient has MRSA on his skin only, then they will require decolonisation treatment, which involves antibacterial cream, antibacterial shampoo and daily separate laundry washes. If the patient has an MRSA infection, then antibiotics will usually be indicated.

STATION 1.8: BODY MASS INDEX

SCENARIO

Mr Judge is a 49-year-old man who is new to your primary care practice. To complete your records, you wish to have an up-to-date measure of his BMI. Please assess the patient's BMI and relay your findings.

OBJECTIVE

- Assessing BMI

GENERAL ADVICE

- Before assessing a patient's BMI, it is important to ensure he understands what this involves and why you wish to perform the measurement.
- Obtain consent.

EQUIPMENT

- Calibrated scales
- Calibrated ruler

ASSESSING BMI

1. Introduce yourself to the patient and obtain.
2. Ask the patient to remove shoes and all outer clothing (keeping underwear on).
3. Weigh the patient using calibrated scales.
4. Measure the patient's height using a calibrated ruler, asking him to stand straight.
5. Calculate the BMI using the following formula:

$$BMI = \frac{Weight\ in\ Kilograms(Kg)}{Height\ in\ metres(m)^2}$$

6. Document your findings and discuss them with the patient.

Interpreting BMI

BMI	WEIGHT STATUS
<18.5	Underweight
18.5–24.9	Expected range
25–29.9	Overweight
>30	Obese

Present Your Findings

Today I measured the weight and height of Mr Judge, a 49-year-old man: this was 90 kg and 1.7 m, respectively. His BMI was calculated to be 31.1, suggesting that he is obese. I have discussed this finding with the patient, informed him of the risks associated with obesity and signposted him to weight loss services. I would also like to take a detailed history and assess his cardiovascular risk.

QUESTIONS AND ANSWERS FOR CANDIDATE

What might you measure instead if you were unable to measure the patient's height?
- If this is not possible, you can either substitute the height with an estimate or use ulnar length to calculate height (conversion tables for this can be found online).

Mark Scheme for Examiner

	0	1	2	3
Introduction and General Preparation				
Introduces self and washes hands				
Confirms patient's identity with three points of identification				
Explains procedure, identifies concerns and obtains consent				
Assessing BMI				
Asks the patient to remove outer clothing				
Weighs the patient				
Measures the patient's height				
Correctly calculates BMI				
Finishing				
Thanks the patient for his time, and gives the patient privacy to get dressed again if required				
Documents findings in patient notes				
Discusses findings with patient				

0 = Not attempted
1 = Performed, with room for improvement
2 = Adequately performed
3 = Performed beyond level expected

Name some medical causes of obesity.
- Endocrine disorders; for example, Cushing's syndrome, hypothyroidism
- Genetic disorders; for example, Prader–Willi syndrome
- Iatrogenic; for example, steroids

Name three cancers for which being overweight is a risk factor.
- Oesophageal
- Stomach
- Bowel
- Liver
- Pancreas
- Gallbladder
- Breast
- Uterus
- Ovary
- Kidney
- Thyroid
- Myeloma
- Meningioma

In which groups of people might the BMI be misleading?
- Patients with a high muscle mass; for example, athletes
- Pregnant patients

What simple lifestyle changes might help manage obesity?
- Increasing amount of physical activity
- Eating a balanced healthy diet
- Reducing the amount of mental stress
- Getting enough sleep

 Tip Box

BMI is a screening tool and is not diagnostic. It can assist healthcare professionals in identifying possible weight problems in adults.

 Fact Box

Waist size is also a good additional measurement to take into account to assess if someone is carrying an excessive amount of abdominal fat, which can increase their risk of various conditions such as heart disease, type 2 diabetes and stroke.

STATION 1.9: NUTRITIONAL ASSESSMENT

SCENARIO

Mr Moran is a 72-year-old man with dementia from a nursing home. He has been on the ward for several days for the management of pneumonia and a urinary tract infection. Your registrar has asked you to perform a nutritional assessment.

OBJECTIVES

- Become competent at using the Malnutrition Universal Screening Tool (MUST)
- Become competent at managing malnutrition

GENERAL ADVICE

- Obtain consent.
- Explain to the patient about the questions you are about to ask him.
- Use the MUST to assess the patient's nutrition.
- In this case, the patient has dementia so you may need to speak to family and other health-care professionals to obtain the information you require.

MUST SCREENING TOOL

MUST is a screening tool used to identify adults who are malnourished, at risk of malnutrition or obese.

MUST SCREENING TOOL

Step 1 Calculate BMI	Step 2 Weight loss score	Step 3 Acute disease effect score	Step 4 Overall risk of malnutrition (add together the scores for steps 1–3)
0: BMI >20 kg/m^2	0: <5% unplanned weight loss in the past 3–6 months	2: If the patient has been acutely ill and there has been no nutritional intake for >5 days	0 = Low risk Repeat MUST weekly Weigh weekly
1: BMI >18.5–20 kg/m^2	1: 5–10% unplanned weight loss in the past 3–6 months		1 = Medium risk Start nutrition action plan Repeat MUST weekly Weigh weekly
2: BMI <18.5 kg/m^2	2: >10% unplanned weight loss in the past 3–6 months		2 = High risk Refer to dietician PLUS As for medium risk

Managing Problems with Nutrition

SIMPLE MEASURES
- Refer to dietician
- Ensure the medical team is aware of patients with nutritional problems
- Follow trust protocol for managing patients with nutritional problems

DIETARY SUPPLEMENTATION
- High-energy drinks
- Full-fat milk
- Multivitamins

ALTERNATIVE METHODS OF FEEDING
- Nasogastric (NG) tubing: Indicated in those who cannot eat or drink normally by mouth (for example, those with an 'unsafe' swallow)
- Total parenteral nutrition/IV feeding: Indicated when the gastrointestinal tract is non-functional (for example, in short-bowel syndrome)

Mark Scheme for Examiner

	0	1	2	3
Introduction and General Preparation				
Introduces self and washes hands				
Confirms patient's identity with three points of identification				
Explains procedure, identifies concerns and obtains consent				
Assessing Nutrition Status				
Calculates BMI				
Discusses any weight loss (and, if appropriate, the time frame)				
Discusses acute disease and nutritional intake				
Calculates risk of malnutrition				

Continued

Mark Scheme for Examiner—cont'd

	0	1	2	3
Finishing				
Thanks the patient for his time				
Documents findings in the patient notes				
Discusses the findings with the patient				

0 = Not attempted
1 = Performed, with room for improvement
2 = Adequately performed
3 = Performed beyond level expected

? QUESTIONS AND ANSWERS FOR CANDIDATE

Give four risk factors that can predispose to malnutrition.

- Swallowing problems; for example, stroke or motor neurone disease
- Psychological disease; for example, depression, dementia
- Malabsorption; for example, coeliac disease, inflammatory bowel disease
- Chronic illness; for example, chronic obstructive pulmonary disease (COPD) resulting in increased energy demands
- Lack of education, learning difficulties or poor access to food
- Acute illness resulting in increased energy demands and often reduced oral intake

What investigations would you consider undertaking in a patient who is malnourished?

- Haematological studies
- Serum albumin
- Retinol-binding protein
- Prealbumin
- Transferrin
- Creatinine
- Blood urea nitrogen (BUN)

Apart from doctors, which other healthcare professionals would you include in the management of a malnourished patient?

- Dieticians
- Nurses
- Home carer visitors
- Occupational therapists
- If appropriate, psychiatrists
- If appropriate, social workers
- If appropriate, speech and language therapists

When performing a nutrition-focused physical examination, what features are important to note?

- BMI
- Nail signs; for example, clubbing, leukonychia, koilonychia
- Peripheral oedema
- Muscle wasting
- Subcutaneous fat loss
- Ascites
- Loose skin
- Presence of nutritional assistance or supplements
- Vital signs
- Glossitis and angular stomatitis
- Gingivitis
- Bowed legs

What are the two classical clinical presentations of protein malnutrition?

- Kwashiorkor is a severe form of malnutrition due to lack of protein and other essential vitamins and minerals. It is more common in low income countries and affects children more than adults. Patients usually present with oedema beginning in the legs, loss of muscle mass and an enlarged abdomen ('pot belly'), and are very susceptible to infections.
- Marasmus is another severe form of malnutrition that, again, affects children more than adults. Patients typically present with thinness and loss of muscle and fat without any signs of oedema.

 Tip Box

Mid upper-arm circumference can be used as an alternative to estimate a patient's BMI category.

 Fact Box

The most common cause of malnutrition in children is long-term diseases such as cystic fibrosis, congenital heart disease and cerebral palsy.

GUIDELINES

BAPEN, 2022. Malnutrition Universal Screening Tool. https://www.bapen.org.uk/screening-and-must/must-calculator.

Blood Tests

Outline

STATION 2.1: VENEPUNCTURE/ PHLEBOTOMY

SCENARIO

Mr Fredrick is a 50-year-old man who is attending your clinic for a repeat blood test to check his haemoglobin, having recently been in hospital and having received a blood transfusion. Please explain to him what you are going to do, and then demonstrate how you would take blood on the mannequin provided.

OBJECTIVES

- To learn the correct techniques for phlebotomy
- To learn the common blood tests and draw order

GENERAL ADVICE

1. Check patient identification and obtain consent.
2. Check whether the patient has any allergies.
3. Check whether the patient is needle-phobic.
4. Check for any issues that may affect selection of the site of phlebotomy; for example, whether he has lymphoedema or an arteriovenous fistula, or (if female) has had a mastectomy.

EQUIPMENT CHECKLIST

(Remember to check expiry dates on all equipment [Fig. 2.1].)
- Tray: Either single-use, disposable sterilised tray or a decontaminated plastic tray that is cleaned pre-/post-procedure
- Single-use disposable apron
- Non-sterile gloves
- Disposable tourniquet
- Skin-cleansing solution (2% chlorhexidine and 70% isopropyl alcohol [for example, ChloraPrep])
- Venepuncture needle
- Vacutainer

- Blood bottles
- Cotton wool
- Tape
- Sharps bin: The sharps bin should always be taken to the point of care.

Note: Skin-cleansing solutions and method will vary depending on local policy. If taking blood cultures, blood culture bottle ports will need to be fully cleaned and allowed to dry fully before use.

EXPLAINING VENEPUNCTURE TO THE PATIENT

1. We need to take a blood sample.
2. We need to put a tight band around your arm to 'bring up' the vein.
3. A small needle is placed into one of your veins in the arm.
4. It will be slightly painful.
5. A blood sample will then be taken.
6. It is possible the doctor may be unable to take a blood sample at the first attempt. If this happens, the doctor will ask your permission before trying again.

PERFORMING VENEPUNCTURE

- Clean hands, don non-sterile gloves and apply a single-use disposable apron (Fig. 2.2).
- Place the tourniquet 7–10 cm proximal to the proposed insertion point (Fig. 2.3).
- Select the vein. The vein should feel 'bouncy'—if not, it is either inadequately filled or, if rigid, it may be thrombosed.
- Loosen the tourniquet.
- Clean the site. Clean for 30 seconds with ChloraPrep with an up-and-down, back-and-forth friction technique. Allow to dry completely (Fig. 2.4).
- Retighten the tourniquet. Attach the venepuncture needle to the Vacutainer.
- Puncture the vein using a non-touch technique (NTT), warning the patient of a 'sharp scratch' (Fig. 2.5).

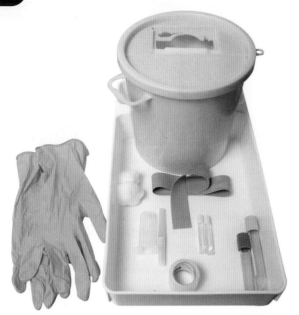

Fig. 2.1 Ensure you have all the equipment you require before heading to the bedside.

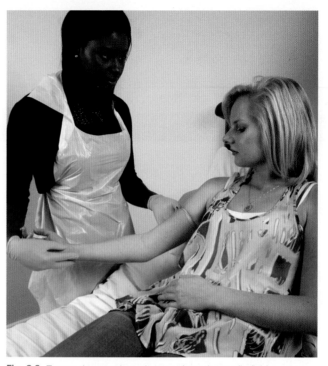

Fig. 2.3 Ensure the tourniquet is away from the sterile field.

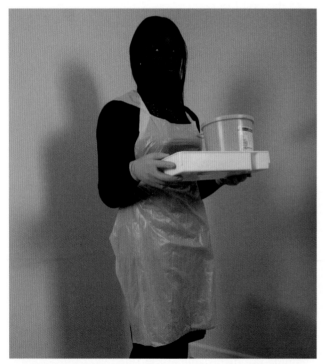

Fig. 2.2 Correctly prepare for the procedure using appropriate personal protective equipment (PPE).

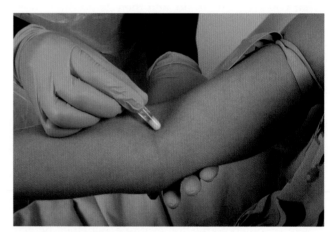

Fig. 2.4 Ensure skin is clean.

- Draw blood by attaching bottles to the Vacutainer, then invert the bottles.
- Release the tourniquet.
- Immediately dispose of all sharps (Fig. 2.6).

- Apply pressure to the puncture site with cotton wool for 2 min or until bleeding stops.
- Secure with tape (Fig. 2.7).
- Label the bottles at the bedside (Fig. 2.8).
- Inform the patient to let a member of staff know if the site is painful, continues to bleed, or if the patient has any other concerns.
- Explain that they can remove the dressing after a couple of hours.

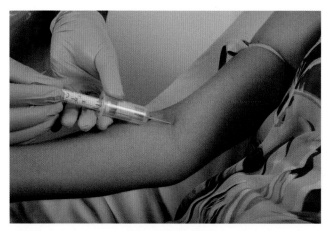

Fig. 2.5 Make sure you collect blood in the order of draw.

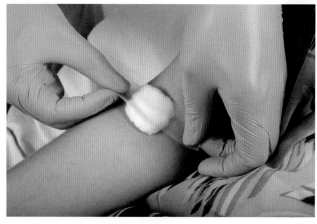

Fig. 2.7 Ask the patient to apply pressure, if they are able to.

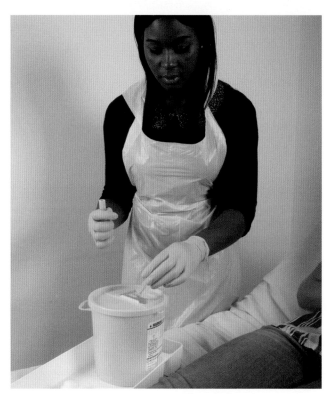

Fig. 2.6 Take the sharps bin to the bedside with you.

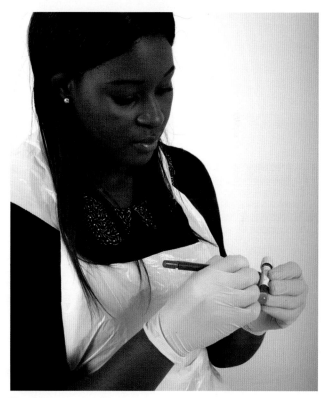

Fig. 2.8 Correctly label the bottles at the bedside.

FINISHING

- Dispose of equipment.
- Clean the tray.
- Dispose of gloves and wash your hands.
- Send the samples to the pathology laboratory.
- Document the procedure.

DOCUMENT THE PROCEDURE

Document under the following headings:
- Venepuncture performed
- Date, time and place
- Indications for the procedure
- Patient consent
- Site used
- Number of attempts
- Number of samples sent to the pathology laboratory
- Complications

BLOOD BOTTLES

(In order of draw; note that colours may vary between hospitals).

Tube	Colour/Additive	What it can measure	Number of times to invert
Blood cultures	Blue (aerobic) — 5 mL Purple (anaerobic) — 5 mL	Blood culture and sensitivity	3–4
Light blue	Sodium citrate — 2.7 mL	International normalised ratio (INR), prothrombin time (PT), activated partial thromboplastin time (APTT)	3–4
Red	Plain — 10 mL	Hepatitis status, rubella serology, virology, cancer antigen 125 (CA-125), coeliac screen	5–6
Gold	Serum separating tube (SST) — 5 mL	Thyroid function tests (TFTs), liver function tests (LFTs), hormones, lipids/triglycerides, cholesterol, urea and electrolyte (U&Es), creatine kinase (CK), digoxin levels, paracetamol levels, prostate-specific antigen (PSA), beta-human chorionic gonadotrophin (β-hCG), haematinics, amylase	5–6
Green	Lithium heparin — 6 mL	Amino acids, cortisol, parathyroid hormone (PTH)	8–10
Lavender	Ethylenediaminetetraacetic acid (EDTA) — 3 mL	Full blood count (FBC), HbA_{1c}, human leukocyte antigen (HLA)-B27, cyclosporine, erythrocyte sedimentation rate (ESR)	8–10
Pink	EDTA — 6 mL	Group and save, cross-match, blood group	8–10
Grey	Fluoride oxalate — 2 mL	Glucose, ethanol	8–10
Royal blue	EDTA — 5 mL	Trace elements: Zinc, copper, selenium, manganese, lead	8–10

Mark Scheme for Examiner

	0	1	2	3
Introduction and General Advice				
Introduces self and washes hands				
Confirms patient's identity with three points of identification				
Explains procedure, identifies concerns and obtains consent				
Checks for allergies and needle phobia, and any contraindications to use of left or right arm				
Preparation				
Obtains equipment and checks expiry dates				
Applies single-use apron, washes hands and dons non-sterile gloves				
Assembles equipment				
Drawing Blood				
Applies disposable tourniquet				
Chooses an appropriate vein and loosens the tourniquet				
Cleans puncture site and retightens tourniquet				
Warns patient				
Punctures vein and obtains sample				
Selects correct draw order (if applicable)				
Removes tourniquet				
Removes needle and applies pressure				
Disposes of sharp immediately				
Applies dressing over puncture site				
Finishing				
Tells patient to inform staff if site becomes painful or continues to bleed and that they can remove the dressing after a few hours				
Labels blood bottles at the bedside				
Disposes of equipment and cleans tray				
Removes gloves and wash hands				
Sends blood sample to pathology lab				

Mark Scheme for Examiner—cont'd

	0	1	2	3
General Points				
Talks throughout the procedure to the patient				
Avoids patient contamination (i.e. non-touch technique [NTT])				

0 = Not attempted
1 = Performed, with room for improvement
2 = Adequately performed
3 = Performed beyond level expected

QUESTIONS AND ANSWERS FOR CANDIDATE

What is the order of draw for full blood count (FBC), urea and electrolytes (U&Es) and clotting?

1. Clotting
2. U&Es
3. FBC

Name three causes of hyperkalaemia.

- Drugs; for example, potassium-sparing diuretics, angiotensin-converting enzyme (ACE) inhibitors
- Renal insufficiency (both acute and chronic renal disease may cause hyperkalaemia)
- Diabetic ketoacidosis
- Burns
- Rhabdomyolysis
- Aldosterone deficiency
- Addisonian crises
- Metabolic acidosis

What additives are found in the different blood tubes?

- FBC: Ethylenediaminetetraacetic acid (EDTA)
- Clotting: Citrate
- Plasma analysis: Lithium heparin (or sodium heparin)
- Glucose: Potassium oxalate and sodium fluoride
- Serum tube: No additive, because you want the blood to clot and to centrifuge the serum

How might an FBC help you differentiate between a bacterial and a viral infection?

- White cell count (WCC) is usually raised in an infection.
- In a bacterial infection, you usually see an increase in neutrophils and decrease in lymphocytes.
- In a viral infection, you usually see an increase in lymphocytes and decrease in neutrophils.

What is CK, and when would you request it?

- CK stands for creatine kinase, also known as creatine phosphokinase (CPK). This is an enzyme that is present in all muscle tissues and is released if there is damage to the muscle.
- This is usually indicated if you suspect musculoskeletal or heart disease.

Tip Box

Always fill the coagulation bottle right up to the line; it won't get processed otherwise!

Fact Box

If simultaneously there is both folate and B_{12} deficiency, replace B_{12} first and then folate.

STATION 2.2: BLOOD CULTURES

SCENARIO

Mr London is a 68-year-old man who has recently undergone a laparoscopic right hemicolectomy. He is now 2 days post-op and the staff nurse looking after him has informed you that his temperature is 38.7°C. Your registrar has asked you to take blood cultures from the patient.

OBJECTIVE

- To learn how to take blood cultures

GENERAL ADVICE

1. Ensure that your patient has given consent for the procedure. Ideally, blood cultures should be taken before the administration of antibiotics or just before the next dose of antibiotics.
2. Blood cultures must always be obtained from a fresh stab and not from existing cannulae or lines.
3. When a long-term method of access is in place, such as a central or peripherally inserted central catheter (PICC) line, cultures should be obtained from a fresh stab and the long-term line.
4. When blood cultures have been taken, this should be clearly documented in the notes, with information about the date, time, site (including which port in the case of line cultures) and indications.

EQUIPMENT CHECKLIST

(Remember to check expiry dates on all equipment [Fig. 2.9].)

- Tray: Either single-use, disposable sterilised tray, or a decontaminated plastic tray that is cleaned pre-/post-procedure
- Disposable plastic apron

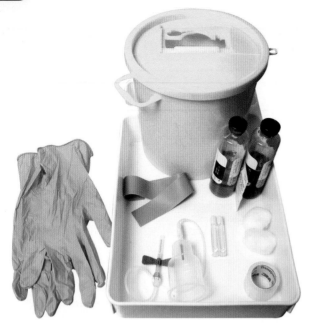

Fig. 2.9 When collecting blood cultures, ensure that the blood bottles are in date.

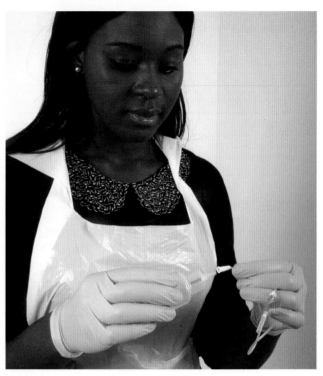

Fig. 2.10 Correctly assemble equipment.

- Non-sterile gloves (or sterile gloves if repalpation of the venepuncture site after cleaning is anticipated)
- Disposable tourniquet
- Skin-cleansing solution; for example, ChloraPrep
- Winged blood collection set
- Blood culture bottle adapter cap
- Aerobic and anaerobic blood culture bottles
- Cotton wool
- Tape
- Sharps bin: The sharps bin should always be taken to the point of care

Note: Skin-cleansing solutions and method will vary depending on local policy.

EXPLAINING THE PROCEDURE TO THE PATIENT

1. We need to take a blood sample to test for any bacteria in your blood because you recently spiked a temperature.
2. We need to put a tight band around your arm to 'bring up' the vein.
3. A small needle is placed into one of your veins in the arm.
4. It will be slightly painful.
5. A blood sample will then be taken into special blood bottles and sent to the laboratory.
6. It is possible the doctor may be unable to take a blood sample at the first attempt. If this happens, the doctor will ask your permission before trying again.

TAKING BLOOD CULTURES

EQUIPMENT PREPARATION

1. Gather the equipment and check the expiry dates of the blood culture bottles.
2. Wash your hands, don gloves and apron.
3. Attach winged blood collection set to blood culture bottle adapted cap (Fig. 2.10).
4. Clean the tops of culture bottles with cleansing preparation. Allow to dry fully.

SKIN PREPARATION

1. Apply disposable tourniquet and palpate to identify a suitable vein.
2. Loosen the tourniquet. Clean the site for 30 seconds with a ChloraPrep swab. Allow to dry fully.
3. Do not repalpate the skin following cleaning.

Note: If a culture is being collected from a central venous catheter, disinfect the access port with a ChloraPrep-impregnated swab.

SAMPLE COLLECTION – WINGED BLOOD COLLECTION SET METHOD

1. Retighten the tourniquet. Warn the patient of a 'sharp scratch'.
2. Insert the needle (bevel up) into the prepared vein.
3. Place the adapter cap over **aerobic** blood collection bottle and pierce the septum (Fig. 2.11).

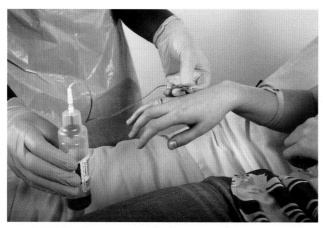

Fig. 2.11 Collect blood into the aerobic bottle first when using a winged blood collection set.

4. Hold the bottle upright and use bottle graduation lines to gauge sample volume accurately.
5. Remove from adapter cap when the correct volume of blood has been collected.
6. Repeat steps 3–5 using the **anaerobic** blood collection bottle.
7. Remove the tourniquet.
8. Remove the winged blood collection set and apply pressure with cotton wool.
9. Dispose of sharps immediately.
10. At the site of the needle puncture, secure cotton wool in place with tape.

11. Label the bottles at the bedside.
12. Inform the patient to let a member of staff know if the site is painful, continues to bleed, or if they have any other concerns.
13. Explain that they can remove the dressing after a couple of hours.
14. Remove gloves and wash hands.
15. Document the procedure in the patient's notes.

FINISHING

- Dispose of equipment.
- Clean the tray.
- Dispose of gloves and wash your hands.
- Send the samples to the pathology laboratory.
- Document the procedure.

DOCUMENT THE PROCEDURE

Document under the following headings:
- Blood culture samples taken
- Date, time and place
- Indications for the procedure
- Patient consent
- Site used
- Number of attempts
- Number of samples sent to the pathology laboratory
- Complications

Mark Scheme for Examiner

	0	1	2	3
Introduction and General Advice				
Introduces self and washes hands				
Confirms patient's identity with three points of identification				
Explains procedure, identifies concerns and obtains consent				
Checks for allergies and needle phobia, and any contraindications to use of left or right arm				
Equipment Preparation				
Obtains equipment and checks expiry dates				
Applies single-use apron, washes hands and dons non-sterile gloves				
Assembles equipment, including attaching winged blood collection set to adapter cap				
Cleans the tops of both culture bottles				
Skin Preparation				
Applies disposable tourniquet. Identifies a suitable vein, then loosens the tourniquet				
Cleans intended puncture site				
Sample Collection – Winged Blood Collection Set Method				
Retightens tourniquet				
Warns patient and then punctures the vein				
Collects blood sample – aerobic first, then anaerobic bottle				
Removes tourniquet				
Removes winged blood collection set and applies pressure over the puncture site				

Continued

Mark Scheme for Examiner—cont'd

	0	1	2	3
Disposes of sharp immediately				
Applies dressing over puncture site				
Finishing				
Tells patient to inform staff if site becomes painful or continues to bleed and that they can remove the dressing after a few hours				
Labels blood bottles at the bedside				
Disposes of equipment and cleans tray				
Removes gloves and washes hands				
Sends blood sample to pathology lab				
Documents procedure in the patient's notes				
General Points				
Talks throughout the procedure to the patient				
Avoids patient contamination (i.e. NTT)				

0 = Not attempted
1 = Performed, with room for improvement
2 = Adequately performed
3 = Performed beyond level expected

❓ QUESTIONS AND ANSWERS FOR CANDIDATE

What signs and symptoms might indicate bacteraemia?
- Core temperature >38°C with or without rigors
- Haemodynamic instability; for example, raised heart rate, lowered blood pressure, reduced urine output, increased capillary refill time (CRT)- note that CRT is less reliable in more pigmented skin.
- Localised symptoms or signs for the source of infection; for example, productive cough and lung crepitations for pneumonia
- Raised respiratory rate and additional signs of respiratory distress; for example, an intercostal recession

For how many days are basic sets of cultures incubated?
- 14 days, with a minimum of 5 days
- This can be longer if bacterial endocarditis is suspected

What are the volumes of blood that are required in different blood culture bottles?
- Aerobic bottle (blue top): Up to 10 mL
- Anaerobic bottle (purple top): Up to 10 mL
- Paediatric bottle (yellow top): Up to 4 mL

What organisms might you suspect in infective endocarditis?
- *Viridans streptococci*
- *Staphylococcus aureu*
- *Haemophilus, Actinobacillus, Cardiobacterium, Eikenella, Kingella* (HACEK) organisms
- *Streptococcus bovis*

What bacteria commonly causes community-acquired pneumonia (CAP)?
- *Streptococcus pneumoniae*
- *Mycoplasma pneumoniae*
- *Chlamydophila pneumoniae*

 Tip Box

If other blood samples are required at the same time as you are taking blood cultures, ensure the blood cultures are taken first before obtaining the remaining samples.

 Fact Box

Standard practice dictates that two sets of blood cultures should be obtained at different times and from different sites, decreasing the possibility of misinterpreting culture results if they become contaminated. If infective endocarditis is suspected, then three sets of blood cultures should be obtained, again from three different sites.

STATION 2.3: ARTERIAL BLOOD GAS

SCENARIO

Mr Bridge is a 57-year-old man who has been admitted due to an exacerbation of his chronic obstructive pulmonary disease (COPD). He is unable to speak in full sentences and has a respiratory rate of 26 breaths/min. He has found no relief from his usual medications. Please perform a radial arterial blood gas (ABG) puncture.

OBJECTIVE

- Performing a radial ABG puncture

GENERAL ADVICE

1. Ensure that your patient has given consent for the procedure.

2. Check whether the patient is on anticoagulant medication.

3. Ideally, the patient would be breathing room air for a minimum of 20 min before the sample is taken. If this is not possible, then we should know what oxygen supplementation (and by extension, the fraction of inspired oxygen [FiO_2]) the patient is receiving, as this needs to be taken into account when interpreting the results.

Allen's Test

This tests the patency of the radial and ulnar arteries, ensuring the circulation to the hand will not be compromised when the radial arterial blood test is performed.

How do you perform the modified Allen's test?

1. Ask the patent to open and close their hand to form a first for 30 s.
2. Whilst the hand is elevated, occlude both the radial and ulnar arteries (Fig. 2.12).
3. While the patient's hand is still elevated, ask the patient to open the hand, which should be pale.
4. Release pressure from the ulnar artery and observe any colour changes.

A normal negative result: Hand colour returns within 5–10 s, suggesting good ulnar artery supply. The radial arterial blood sampling can therefore be safely performed.

An abnormal positive result: Hand colour does not return within 5–10 s, suggesting poor ulnar artery supply. The radial arterial blood sampling cannot be safely performed from this arm.

- Skin-cleansing solution (for example, ChloraPrep)
- ABG set (these vary between trusts)
- Sterile cotton wool
- Tape
- Sharps bin: Sharps bin should always be taken to the point of care

Note: Skin-cleansing solutions and method will vary depending on local policy.

EXPLAINING THE PROCEDURE TO THE PATIENT

1. We need to take a blood sample from your wrist.
2. It will be slightly painful.
3. We will analyse it straight away and it will give us valuable information on the level of different gases in your blood.
4. It is possible the doctor may be unable to take a blood sample at the first attempt. If this happens, the doctor will ask your permission before trying again.

PERFORMING A RADIAL ARTERIAL BLOOD GAS PUNCTURE

SKIN PREPARATION

1. Wash hands and put on non-sterile gloves and apron.
2. Clean site for 30 s with a ChloraPrep swab with an up-and-down, back-and-forth friction technique. Allow to dry fully.

EQUIPMENT CHECKLIST

(Remember to check expiry dates on all equipment [Fig. 2.13].)

- Tray: Either single-use, disposable sterilised tray or a decontaminated plastic tray that is cleaned pre-/post-procedure
- Non-sterile gloves and single-use apron

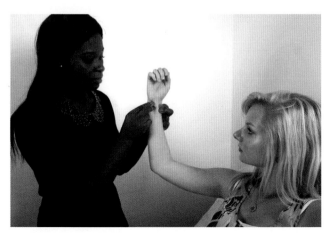

Fig. 2.12 The doctor is occluding both the radial and ulnar arteries.

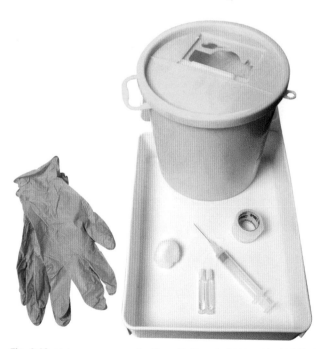

Fig. 2.13 Make sure you are familiar with the arterial blood test kit that is used in your trust.

PALPATING THE RADIAL ARTERY

1. Ensure that the patient is comfortable, with their forearm resting on a flat surface.
2. Hyperextend the wrist joint over a rolled towel.
3. Palpate the radial artery using your index and middle fingers to determine a good position for the procedure.

SAMPLE COLLECTION

Method A

1. Once the radial artery is located, shift your index and middle fingers proximally by 1–2 cm.
2. Hold the needle like a pencil, bevel up.
3. Insert the needle at 45° just distal to your index finger (Fig. 2.14).
4. Advance the needle into the radial artery.
5. Obtain the sample (usually 3 mL).
6. Withdraw the needle.
7. Apply pressure to the puncture site using cotton wool and secure with tape.
8. Direct pressure should be continued until bleeding has stopped.
9. Dispose of the needle in a sharps bin.
10. Gently mix the sample by inverting the syringe up and down.
11. Inform the patient to let a member of staff know if the site is painful, continues to bleed, or if they have any other concerns.
12. Explain that they can remove the dressing after a couple of hours.
13. Take the blood sample to the nearest blood gas analyser.

14. Once analysed, dispose of the syringe into a sharps bin.
15. Remove gloves and wash hands.
16. Document the procedure and findings in the patient's notes.

Method B

1. Once the radial artery is located, separate your index and middle fingers by 2–4 cm.
2. Hold the needle like a pencil, bevel up.
3. Insert the needle at 45° between your index and middle fingers (Fig. 2.15).
4. Perform steps 4–16 as above.

FINISHING

- Dispose of equipment.
- Clean the tray.
- Dispose of gloves and wash your hands.
- Send the samples to the pathology laboratory.
- Document the procedure.

DOCUMENT THE PROCEDURE

Document under the following headings:
- Arterial blood sample taken
- Date, time and place
- Indications for the procedure
- Patient consent
- Modified Allen's test performed
- Site used
- Number of attempts
- Complications
- Results from the sample

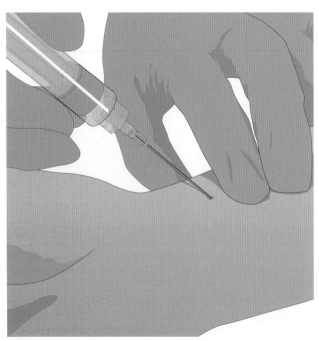

Fig. 2.14 Method A: The ABG needle is inserted distal to the index finger.

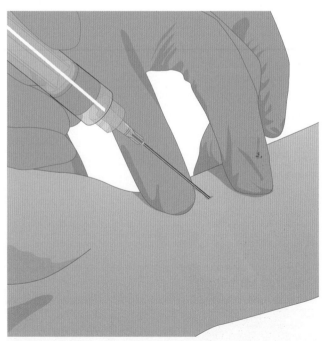

Fig. 2.15 Method B: The ABG needle is inserted between the palpating fingers.

Mark Scheme for Examiner

	0	1	2	3
Introduction and General Advice				
Introduces self and washes hands				
Confirms patient's identity with three points of identification				
Explains procedure, identifies concerns and obtains consent				
Notes respiratory support				
Equipment Preparation				
Obtains equipment and checks expiry dates				
Skin Preparation				
Washes hands and dons non-sterile gloves/apron				
Cleans puncture site				
Palpating the Radial Artery				
Positions the patient's wrist				
Locates puncture site				
Sample Collection				
Punctures the skin to collect the sample (3 mL)				
Removes the needle and applies direct pressure				
Disposes of needle immediately				
Gently mixes the sample				
Applies dressing over puncture site				
Finishing				
Tells patient to inform staff if site becomes painful or continues to bleed and that they can remove the dressing after a few hours				
Disposes of equipment and cleans tray				
Takes sample to nearest blood gas analyser				
Removes gloves/apron and washes hands				
Documents procedure in the patient's notes				
General Points				
Talks throughout the procedure to the patient				
Avoids patient contamination (i.e. NTT)				

0 = Not attempted
1 = Performed, with room for improvement
2 = Adequately performed
3 = Performed beyond level expected

❓ QUESTIONS AND ANSWERS FOR CANDIDATE

What is the normal range for $PaCO_2$?
- 4.7–6.0 kPa

Name three causes of a high anion gap metabolic acidosis.
- Diabetic ketoacidosis
- Lactic acidosis
- Uraemia
- Aspirin overdose

What clinical signs or symptoms might be associated with respiratory distress?
- Increased respiratory rate
- Cyanosis
- Grunting
- Wheezing
- Nasal flaring
- Sweatiness
- Tripod position
- Intercostal retraction

What is type 1 respiratory failure?
- Type 1 respiratory failure is defined as hypoxaemia (PaO_2 <8 kPa) with a low or normal level of carbon dioxide in the blood.

What is type 2 respiratory failure?
- Type 2 respiratory failure is defined as hypoxaemia (PaO_2 <8 kPa) associated with hypercapnia ($PaCO_2$ >6 kPa).

 Tip Box

If filling stops before the syringe is full, retract the needle slightly. Most commonly, this occurs because the needle has pierced the posterior arterial wall, preventing further filling. By retracting the needle, the bevel will be placed inside the artery, allowing filling to occur. Most blood gas analysis machines only require 1 mL of blood.

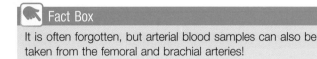

Fact Box

It is often forgotten, but arterial blood samples can also be taken from the femoral and brachial arteries!

STATION 2.4: BLOOD GAS INTERPRETATION

SCENARIO

Mr Bridge is a 57-year-old man who has been admitted due to an exacerbation of his COPD. He is unable to speak in full sentences and has a respiratory rate of 26 breaths/min. He has found no relief from his usual medications. An ABG has been performed. Please discuss the findings with your examiner.

OBJECTIVE

- Interpreting an ABG

GENERAL ADVICE

It is important to know what, if any, ventilatory support or oxygenation the patient is receiving at the time of the ABG sample collection as this will help you to interpret the results.

This might include:
- Percentage of oxygen being supplied
- Type of oxygen mask being used
- Pressure of non-invasive/invasive ventilatory support

Note: Commonly the units for partial pressure are kiloPascals (kPa). However, it can be measured in mmHg. Please ensure that you are familiar with the units and reference ranges used in your hospital.

ABG MEASURES	ABG CALCULATES
PaO$_2$	Base excess (BE)
PaCO$_2$	Anion gap
Arterial oxygen saturation (SaO$_2$)	
pH	
Haemoglobin (Hb)	
Sodium (Na$^+$), potassium (K$^+$),	
calcium (Ca^{2+}), chloride (Cl$^-$),	
lactate, bicarbonate (HCO$_3^-$)	

Normal Blood Gas Ranges (for a patient breathing room air)

Reading	Normal range
pH	7.35–7.45
PaO$_2$	10.6–13.3 kPa
PaCO$_2$	4.7–6.0 kPa
HCO$_3^-$	22–28 mmol/L
Base excess	−2 to +2
SaO$_2$	95%–100%

METHODS FOR INTERPRETING BLOOD GAS RESULTS

ASSESS THE PH

- Low (<7.35) indicates acidosis.
- High (>7.45) indicates alkalosis.

IS THE PH EXPLAINED BY THE PaCO$_2$?

CO$_2$ is an acidic gas. This means that:
- **High levels of CO$_2$** in the blood will cause the blood pH to be **acidotic**.
- **Low levels of CO$_2$** in the blood will cause the blood pH to be **alkalotic**.

For example, if the pH indicated acidosis and the CO$_2$ levels were high, this would imply that the acidosis was due to the excess CO$_2$, and therefore the cause of the acidosis was respiratory.

If the pH indicated acidosis and the CO$_2$ levels were low, this would imply that the cause of the acidosis was *not* respiratory, therefore further questions would need to be asked (see below).

IF THE PH IS NOT EXPLAINED BY THE PaCO$_2$, IS IT EXPLAINED BY THE HCO$_3^-$?

HCO$_3^-$ is alkaline and acts as a buffer. This means that:
- **Low levels of HCO$_3^-$** in the blood indicate **acidosis** as it is 'consumed' in the setting of metabolic acidosis.
- **High levels of HCO$_3^-$** in the blood will cause the blood pH to be **alkalotic**.

For example, if the pH indicated acidosis and the HCO$_3^-$ levels were low, this would imply that the acidosis was explained by the HCO$_3^-$ and therefore the cause of the acidosis was metabolic.

Other important things that should not be ignored when interpreting an ABG result are: PaO$_2$, K$^+$ and Hb levels.

Type of abnormality	pH	PaCO$_2$	HCO$_3^-$	Compensation	Causes		

Respiratory acidosis	↓	↑	↔	↑HCO$_3^-$	• Hypoventilation
					• Lung pathology:
					  - Asthma
					  - COPD
					• Pneumonia
					• Pulmonary oedema
					• Pulmonary embolus
					• Obesity
					• Myasthenia gravis
					• Guillain Barre syndrome
					• Chest wall defects
					• Pharmacological:
					  - Opioids
					  - Sedatives		

Respiratory alkalosis	↑	↓	↔	↓HCO$_3^-$	• Hyperventilation • Stroke • Intracranial bleed • Meningitis		
Metabolic acidosis	↓	↔	↓	↓CO$_2$	*Causes of a high anion gap:* • Diabetic ketoacidosis (DKA) • Lactic acidosis • Uraemia • Aspirin overdose	*Causes of a normal anion gap:* • Diarrhoea • Addison's disease • Renal tubular acidosis • Pancreatic fistula	*Causes of a low anion gap:* • Hypoalbuminaemia • Multiple myeloma
Metabolic alkalosis	↑	↔	↑	↑CO$_2$	• Diarrhoea • Vomiting • Conn's syndrome • Burns • Hypokalaemia		

WORKED EXAMPLES

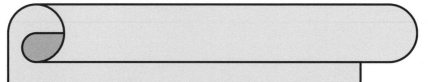

Request No:	24891022	**Patient No:**	4616
Date:	27.11.2013	**DOB:**	27.03.1959
Time:	01:48		

At 37°C   **Arterial Ref Range**

pH..................	7.28	7.35-7.45
pCO_2.............	8.1	4.7-6.0
pO_2...............	12.2	10.6-13.3
FiO_2..............	0.21	
Cl^-..................	100	95-105
Na^+.................	142	135-145
K^+...................	3.3	3.5-5.0
HCO_3^-	25	22-28

❗ Example 1

pH 7.28	Is the pH acidotic or alkalotic?	Acidotic
$PaCO_2$ 8.1	Is the pH explained by the $PaCO_2$?	Yes
HCO_3^- 25	Is the pH explained by the HCO_3^-?	No
	Is there evidence of compensation?	No

- The HCO_3^- level is normal
- The pH is abnormal (so no evidence of full compensation)

Interpretation: Respiratory acidosis with no compensation (for example, more likely an acute attack)

Request No:	60350029	**Patient No:**	1490
Date:	20.12.2013	**DOB:**	21.08.1971
Time:	07:51		

At 37°C		**Arterial Ref Range**
pH..................	7.48	7.35-7.45
pCO$_2$.............	8.4	4.7-6.0
pO$_2$...............	11.8	10.6-13.3
FiO$_2$..............	0.21	
Cl$^-$..................	101	95-105
Na$^+$.................	136	135-145
K$^+$....................	4.2	3.5-5.0
HCO$_3^-$	38	22-28

! Example 2

pH 7.48	Is the pH acidotic or alkalotic?	Alkalotic
PaCO$_2$ 8.4	Is the pH explained by the PaCO$_2$?	No
HCO$_3^-$ 38	Is the pH explained by the HCO$_3^-$?	Yes
	Is there evidence of compensation?	Yes
		• The PaCO$_2$ level is abnormal (implying compensation)
		• The pH is abnormal (so no evidence of full compensation)

Interpretation: Metabolic alkalosis with partial respiratory compensation

Request No:	6036781	Patient No:	8912
Date:	20.02.2014	DOB:	01.04.1939
Time:	13:56		

At 37°C		Arterial Ref Range
pH.................	7.30	7.35-7.45
pCO_2.............	4.1	4.7-6.0
pO_2...............	13.2	10.6-13.3
FiO_2..............	0.21	
Cl^-.................	99	95-105
Na^+.................	137	135-145
K^+...................	3.;1	3.5-5.0
HCO_3^-	18	22-28

 Example 3

pH 7.30	Is the pH acidotic or alkalotic?	Acidotic
$PaCO_2$ 4.1	Is the pH explained by the $PaCO_2$?	No
HCO_3^- 18	Is the pH explained by the HCO_3^-?	Yes
	Is there evidence of compensation?	Yes

- The $PaCO_2$ level is abnormal (implying compensation)
- The pH is abnormal (so no evidence of full compensation)

Interpretation: Metabolic acidosis with partial compensation and an increased anion gap

At 37°C		Arterial Ref Range
Request No: 12569028		**Patient No:** 3337
Date: 01.10.2013		**DOB:** 06.08.1965
Time: 09.03		
pH.................	7.36	7.35-7.45
pCO_2.............	7.9	4.7-6.0
pO_2...............	7.4	10.6-13.3
FiO_2..............	0.21	
Cl^-.................	98	95-105
Na^+.................	136	135-145
K^+....................	4.0	3.5-5.0
HCO_3^-	34	22-28

❗ Mr Bridge's results

pH 7.36	Is the pH acidotic or alkalotic?	Normal (but almost acidotic)
$PaCO_2$ 7.9	Is the pH explained by the $PaCO_2$?	Yes (as pH almost classified as acidotic)
HCO_3^- 34	Is the pH explained by the HCO_3^-?	No
	Is there evidence of compensation?	Yes
		• The HCO_3^- level is normal (implying compensation)
		• The pH is normal (so evidence of full compensation)
PaO_2 6.8	Is the PaO_2 within the normal range?	No
		• The PaO_2 is low, indicating hypoxaemia

ASSESSING OTHER ANALYTES

An arterial sample can provide a rapid indication of important analytes such as K^+, Hb and lactate. This can assist in diagnosis and guide early intervention. These can also be obtained from a venous blood gas (VBG).

ASSESSING OXYGENATION AND VENTILATION

Why is it important to look at the PaO_2?

• The PaO_2 gives an indication of oxygen uptake. When assessing the PaO_2, it is vital to consider the $PaCO_2$ at the same time.

Respiratory failure: type 1 — failure to oxygenate
• Characterised by: $PaO_2 < 8$ kPa and $PaCO_2 =$ normal/low
Respiratory failure: type 2 — failure to ventilate
• Characterised by: $PaO_2 < 8$ kPa and $PaCO_2 > 6$ kPa

COMPENSATION

• When there has been deviation from the normal blood pH, the body activates pathways to try to compensate for the deviation and attempts to bring the pH back within the normal range.
• The lungs compensate for a metabolic disturbance by altering the levels of carbon dioxide—this is generally rapid and can occur within minutes.

- The kidneys compensate for a respiratory disturbance by controlling the levels of bicarbonate ions — this is generally slower and takes from a few days to a week to occur.
- A patient can be uncompensated — this usually implies an acute event, where the body has not had time to adapt to the change in pH.
- A patient can be partially compensated — this implies the pH is out of the normal range and the body is making an attempt to compensate for the disturbance. For example, there may be a respiratory acidosis (raised carbon dioxide), and a small metabolic alkalosis (raised bicarbonate) to compensate. However, the compensation is only partial, and therefore the patient remains acidotic.
- A patient can be fully compensated — this implies the pH is now within the normal range but other values are still abnormal in order to correct the underlying disturbance. This implies a chronic process.

Note: It is important to remember that, in general, overcompensation does not happen. The body brings the pH back within the normal range.

Present Your Findings

Mr Bridge's results show borderline respiratory acidosis with full metabolic compensation and concurrent hypoxia. Putting it all together, this is most likely chronic type 2 respiratory failure with renal compensation. I would like to discuss with a senior to decide whether the patient should aim for a lower oxygen requirement of 88%—92%, and whether he requires additional respiratory support.

Mark Scheme for Examiner

	0	1	2	3
Introduction and General Preparation				
Introduces self and washes hands				
Confirms patient's identity on blood gas reading				
Checks if patient has respiratory support; for example, ventilation or oxygenation				
Checks units used				
Interpreting Results				
Discusses pH				
Discusses pH and $PaCO_2$				
Discuses pH and HCO_3^-				
Discusses PaO_2, metabolites and haemoglobin				
If relevant, discusses anion gap				
If relevant, discusses compensation				
Finishing				
Discusses topic logically				
Concludes findings				
Discusses causes for blood gas results				
Discusses management of patient				
Documents results and management plan in the patient's notes				
Discusses findings with patient				

0 = Not attempted
1 = Performed, with room for improvement
2 = Adequately performed
3 = Performed beyond level expected

❓ QUESTIONS AND ANSWERS FOR CANDIDATE

What is the normal range for PaCO₂?
- 4.7–6.0 kPa

Name three causes of a high anion gap metabolic acidosis.
- Diabetic ketoacidosis (DKA)
- Lactic acidosis
- Uraemia
- Aspirin overdose

Discuss the hypoxic drive found in patients with chronic type 2 respiratory failure.
- Normally, carbon dioxide is the main stimulus for the respiratory drive. An individual who is a chronic carbon dioxide retainer, for example, some COPD patients, may have inefficient gaseous exchange, leading to a chronic state of hypercapnia.
- This shifts the patient from a normal respiratory drive to a hypoxic drive, which is why their target pulse oximetry is 88%–92%.

Name three causes of type 1 respiratory failure.
Type 1 respiratory failure occurs because of damage to the lung tissue. This can be seen in:
- Pulmonary oedema
- Pneumonia
- Acute respiratory distress syndrome (ARDS)
- Chronic pulmonary fibrosis
- Pneumothorax
- Pulmonary embolism (PE)

Name three causes of type 2 respiratory failure.
Type 2 respiratory failure is caused by inadequate ventilation of the lung tissue. This can be caused by:
- COPD
- Chest wall deformities
- Respiratory muscle weakness; for example, in myasthenia gravis and other muscle disorders
- Obesity

Tip Box

To help you determine the cause of a patient's metabolic acidosis, the anion gap can be calculated:

$$\text{Anion gap} = (Na^+ + K^+) - (Cl^- + HCO_3^-)$$

Normal range 6–16 mmol/L.

Fact Box

Low pH and high CO_2 imply *respiratory acidosis*. High pH and low CO_2 imply *respiratory alkalosis*. Low pH and HCO_3^- imply *metabolic acidosis*. High pH and high HCO_3^- imply *metabolic alkalosis*.

3

Acute Patient Management

Outline

STATION 3.1: IMMEDIATE LIFE SUPPORT

SCENARIO

You are working on a busy gastroenterology ward when you come across an unresponsive patient in one of the side rooms. Approach this mannequin as you would the patient and perform resuscitation as necessary. Follow any instructions that are given by the examiners during this station.

OBJECTIVES

- To recognise a patient in cardiac arrest
- To be able to perform immediate life support (ILS)
- To know the treatment algorithms for shockable and non-shockable rhythms

GENERAL ADVICE

- ILS is commonly tested with the use of a resuscitation mannequin.
- It is crucially important to use a systemic approach when dealing with any critically ill patient.
- 'DRS ABC' is a useful and well-known mnemonic that will allow you to initiate basic life support (BLS) in a systematic and structured manner (see below).

DANGER

Your own safety is vital — look out for any hazards that might put you at risk. Ask: 'Is it safe to approach?'

RESPONSE

Shake the dummy lightly and shout, 'Hello, can you hear me?', whilst applying a painful stimulus.

SHOUT

Shout for help in the event of an unresponsive patient.

AIRWAY

1. If there is no concern about a spinal injury, perform a head tilt, chin lift manoeuvre (Fig. 3.1).
2. Clear the mouth of any obstruction or foreign body if confident that the object can be removed.
3. Use of suction apparatus or repositioning the patient on their side may help (Fig. 3.2).

BREATHING AND CIRCULATION

Simultaneously (whilst maintaining the chin lift):
- **Look** for chest movement for 10 s
- **Listen** for breath sounds for 10 s
- **Feel** the carotid pulse for 10 s

In clinical practice, if in doubt, call the crash team and start cardiopulmonary resuscitation (CPR):
- You should proceed to chest compressions immediately provided that you are confident further help is on the way. Within hospital, this means putting out a crash call via the switchboard. Send a colleague to perform this if it has not been done already, giving the details of the clinical scenario (adult cardiac arrest) and your location (ward).
- Ask your colleague to bring back the crash trolley on their return — this will contain vital resuscitation equipment.

CHEST COMPRESSION

1. Start chest compressions:
   - **Position:** directly over the bottom half of the sternum (Fig. 3.3)
   - **Rate:** 100–120/min
   - **Depth:** one-third of the depth of the chest. In most adults this equates to 5–6 cm
2. After 30 compressions, give two breaths using a bag valve mask device connected to high-flow oxygen (15 L/min). Make sure you maintain a patient

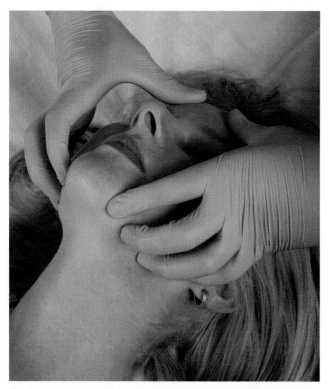

Fig. 3.1 This simple action can sometimes be enough to open an airway.

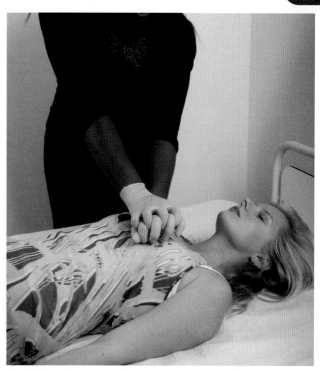

Fig. 3.3 Use both hands to perform compressions on an adult.

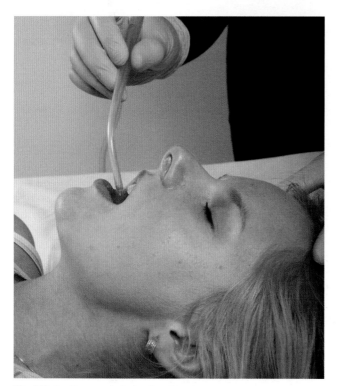

Fig. 3.2 Suction may help to clear the airway.

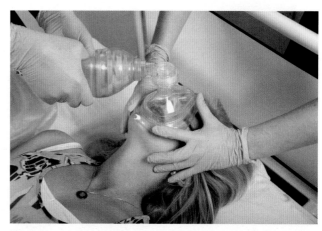

Fig. 3.4 If possible, use two people to operate a bag valve mask.

airway, otherwise bag valve ventilation will not work (Fig. 3.4). The use of airway adjuncts may be required.

3. Continue compressions and breaths at a rate of 30:2.

DEFIBRILLATION

1. Ask your colleague to proceed with the chest compressions and ventilation breaths.

2. Turn on the defibrillator and apply the self-adhesive defibrillation/monitoring pads (ensure that you familiarise yourself with the defibrillators in local use).

3. One pad is placed below the right clavicle, the second is placed in the V6 position in the mid-axillary line on the left (Fig. 3.5).

4. Ensure that chest compressions continue whilst the pads are being sited.

5. Once the pads are connected, charge defibrillator, asking all (except the person performing CPR) to stand clear. Ensure oxygen is moved away. Once charged, ask your helper to stop CPR so that you can assess the rhythm on the defibrillator display (Fig. 3.6).

6. The principal purpose of the rhythm check is to determine whether it is **shockable** or **non-shockable**, and

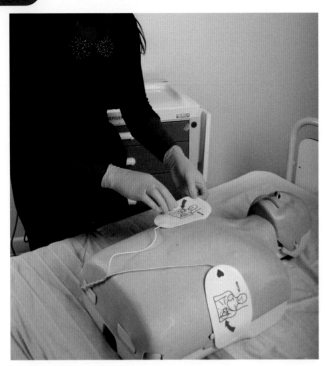

Fig. 3.5 Correct position of the pads is important.

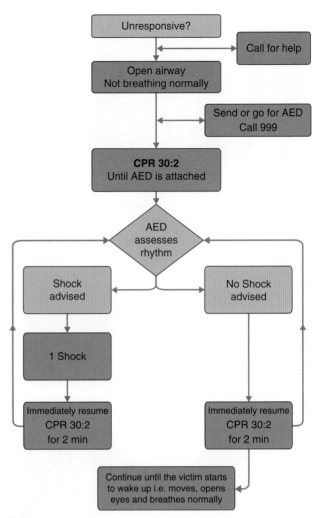

Fig. 3.7 Resuscitation Council (UK) automated external defibrillator (AED) algorithm.

Management of Shockable Rhythms

1. State clearly, 'This is VF/pVT, this is a shockable rhythm'.
2. Ensure that everyone is clear of the patient. Oxygen should be moved away (including oxygen being delivered by a bag valve mask).
3. Press the shock button, stating 'Shocking' just before you do so.
4. Immediately resume chest compressions and ventilation at a ratio of 30:2 for 2 min, without pausing to reassess rhythm and look for signs of life.
5. Just prior to the next rhythm check, charge the defibrillator whilst continuing CPR.
6. At the 2-min mark, cease chest compressions and perform a second rhythm check. Repeat steps 1–6 if still in shockable rhythm.

Drugs Given During Shockable Cardiac Arrest

After the third shock, administer:

- Adrenaline 1 mg intravenously (IV) or interosseously (IO)
- Amiodarone 300 mg IV/IO

After subsequent alternate shocks (every 3–5 min), administer:

- Adrenaline 1 mg IV/IO

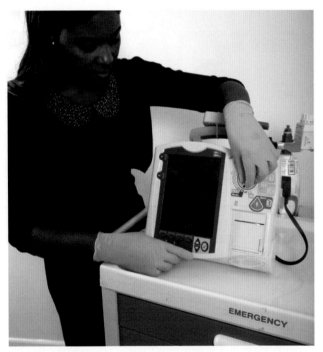

Fig. 3.6 Ensure you are familiar with the defibrillator used in your trust.

manage according to the Resuscitation Council algorithms (Figs. 3.7 and 3.8).

SHOCKABLE RHYTHMS

- Pulseless ventricular tachycardia (pVT) – regular, broad complex tachycardia (Fig. 3.9)
- Ventricular fibrillation (VF) – irregular with varying amplitude and frequency (Fig. 3.10)

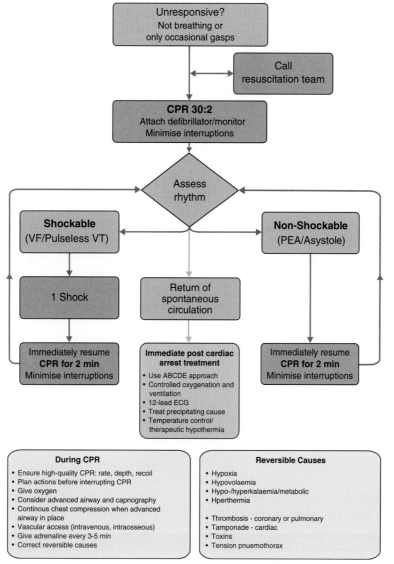

Fig. 3.8 Resuscitation Council (UK) adult advanced life support (if manually assessed). *PEA, pulseless electrical activity.*

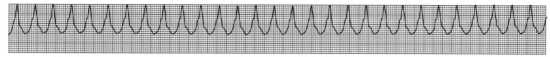

Fig. 3.9 VT rhythm strip.

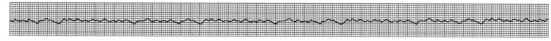

Fig. 3.10 VF rhythm strip.

Amioderone 150 mg IV/IO should be given after the 5th shock.

NON-SHOCKABLE RHYTHMS

- Pulseless electrical activity (PEA) — organised electrical activity but no pulse
- Asystole — no electrical activity

Management of Non-Shockable Rhythms

1. State clearly, 'This is PEA/asystole, this is a non-shockable rhythm.'
2. Press the 'charge dump' button on the defibrillator and recommence chest compressions.
3. Administer 1 mg of adrenaline IV/IO as soon as possible.
4. Proceed with a ratio of 30:2 chest compressions: ventilation breaths.

5. Just before the next 2-min rhythm check, charge the defibrillator whilst continuing CPR.

6. Pause compressions to perform a rhythm check at the 2-min mark.

7. If there is a non-shockable rhythm, dump the charge and recommence chest compressions. Repeat steps 1–7 if still in non-shockable rhythm and no pulse is palpable.

TASKS TO BE PERFORMED DURING RESUSCITATION

AIRWAY

- Consider an advanced airway or supraglottic airway device (for example, an endotracheal (ET) tube or laryngeal mask airway (LMA)), allowing for continuous and simultaneous chest compressions and ventilation.

BREATHING

- Administer high-concentration oxygen.
- Perform a venous blood gas measurement.

CIRCULATION

- Ensure good-quality chest compressions — switch team members every 2 min or sooner, if possible.
- Establish adequate IV access, ideally two large-gauge cannulae. Other methods include IO access.

RECOVERY POSITION

If a patient is unresponsive but breathing normally, then place them into the recovery position (Fig. 3.11).

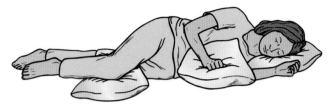

Fig. 3.11 Patient put into the recovery position. (Source: Perry, A. G., Potter, P. A., Ostendorf, W., & Laplante, N. (2022). *Skills Performance Checklists for Clinical Nursing Skills & Techniques*. Elsevier Inc.)

This position keeps the patient's airway open and if the patient were to vomit, the vomit is directed away from the trachea to reduce the possibility of blocking the airway. The following steps guide you through how to place someone into the recovery position:

1. Kneel to one side of the patient and straighten out all of their limbs while the patient is lying supine.
2. If the patient is wearing glasses or has large items in their pockets, remove these.
3. Place the arm closest to you at a right angle to their body, with the elbow flexed and the palm facing upwards to the sky.
4. Then bring the arm of the patient furthest from you across the chest and place the back of their hand against their cheek closest to you. Hold it here for the patient with your hand closest to the patient's head.
5. With your other hand, flex the patient's knee furthest away from you and place that foot on the floor.
6. While keeping the back of the patient's hand against their cheek, pull the far leg at the lateral side of the flexed knee and roll the patient towards you on to their side.

Reversible Causes of Cardiac Arrest

Cause	Management
Hypoxia	You will be giving close to 100% oxygen (O_2) by bag and mask. Once the anaesthetist arrives, they can intubate the patient to secure the airway and ensure optimal oxygenation
Hypovolaemia	Hypovolaemia, of any cause, is managed initially with IV fluids. Inotropes may be required if the patient is not fluid-responsive. Thereafter, management depends upon the cause (for example, antibiotics for septic shock, endoscopy and transfusion for haemorrhage secondary to an upper gastrointestinal bleed (UGIB), etc)
Hypothermia	Bair Hugger and warmed IV fluids. It is unusual for this to be the mechanism behind an arrest in a hospital inpatient
Hypo-/hyperkalaemia (and other metabolic disturbances)	This is assessed on a venous gas. In the case of hyperkalaemia, calcium chloride IV should be administered in order to protect the myocardium, as well as salbutamol, and insulin/dextrose to bring down the potassium
Toxins	Attempt to identify potential toxins — check the patient's notes and ask staff. Treat accordingly (for example, naloxone for opiates)
Thrombosis (coronary or pulmonary)	Follow local guidance for management of acute coronary syndrome and massive pulmonary embolism. Remember that if thrombolysis is used, guidelines state CPR will need to be continued for a minimum of 30 min following this
Tension pneumothorax	Insert a large-bore cannula into the second intercostal space, mid-clavicular line on the affected side and tape in place, inserting a chest drain as definitive management when the patient is stabilised
Cardiac tamponade	Treat with pericardiocentesis

7. Once the patient is on their side, you can adjust the top leg so that it is bent at a right angle.
8. Lastly, gently perform the head tilt, chin lift manoeuvre on the patient so that their airway remains open.

9. Call 999 if this has not already been done, and continue to monitor the patient while waiting for help to arrive.
10. If the patient has stayed in the recovery position for 30 min, roll them into the recovery position on the other side.

Mark Scheme for Examiner

	0	1	2	3
Basic Life Support				
Looks for danger				
Attempts to elicit a response				
Shouts for help				
Checks for airway obstruction. Clears obstruction if possible				
Performs head tilt, chin lift				
Looks for chest rising, feels for pulse, and listens for breath sounds				
Spends no longer than 10 s performing pulse and breathing check				
Puts out cardiac arrest call (instructs colleague or leaves patient, if alone)				
Performs chest compressions correctly (location, rate, depth)				
Performs ventilation breaths correctly				
ILS				
Sites pads correctly. Turns on and charges defibrillator machine (whilst continuing CPR)				
Instructs colleague to stop CPR to assess rhythm				
Shockable Rhythm				
Correctly identifies rhythm as shockable				
Charges defibrillator correctly				
Informs colleague(s) of charging, and instructs those not performing chest compressions to stand clear. Oxygen devices removed				
Instructs colleague performing compressions to stand clear. Delivers shock				
Instructs colleague to resume CPR immediately				
Resumes CPR for 2 min before recharging defibrillator and rechecking rhythm				
Administers adrenaline after 3rd shock and every other shock thereafter, and amiodarone after third and fifth shock				
Non-Shockable Rhythm				
Correctly identifies rhythm as non-shockable				
Immediately instructs colleague to resume CPR and dumps charge				
Does *not* administer shock				
Administers adrenaline immediately				
Resumes CPR for 2 min before recharging defibrillator and rechecking rhythm				
Administers adrenaline every 3–5 min				
During the 2-Minute Cycles				
Mentions or performs IV access Mentions or performs advance airway insertion				
Mentions reversible causes of cardiac arrest				
General Points				
Issues clear commands to colleagues throughout resuscitation attempt				
Maintains situational awareness (checks timing frequently)				

0 = Not attempted
1 = Performed, with room for improvement
2 = Adequately performed
3 = Performed beyond level expected

❓ QUESTIONS AND ANSWERS FOR CANDIDATES

What are the eight reversible causes of cardiac arrest?
These can be remembered as the 4Hs and the 4Ts:
- Hypoxia
- Hypovolaemia
- Hypothermia
- Hyper-/hypokalaemia
- Thrombosis (cardiac/pulmonary)
- Tamponade (cardiac)
- Tension pneumothorax
- Toxins

In the cardiac arrest resuscitation cycle, name the two non-shockable rhythms.
- PEA
- Asystole

When would you administer amiodarone during a resuscitation attempt?
- In the event of a shockable rhythm, after the third and fifth shock has been administered

How does the use of an advanced airway (for example, ET tube) alter the ratio of compression:ventilation breaths?
- Compressions are performed continuously and are only interrupted for rhythm checks/shocks.
- Ventilation breaths are given simultaneously at a rate of 10 breaths/min.

What methods can be used to increase the patient's core body temperature if the patient presented in hypothermia?
- Removal of wet or cold clothes, and moving the patient away from the cold environment
- Covering with blankets and Bair Huggers
- Warmed IV fluid infusion
- Warmed humidified oxygen
- Cavity lavage; for example, gastric, bladder, peritoneal and pleural
- Extracorporeal blood rewarming

 Tip Box

The defibrillator pads contain electrodes for determining cardiac rhythm and are quick to apply — do not waste time attaching electrocardiogram (ECG) electrodes if they are not already on the patient.

 Fact Box

Success of the resuscitation attempt is highly dependent on prompt defibrillation, as well as high-quality CPR and timely arrival of the crash team. Therefore, if you are alone with a patient who you believe is in cardiac arrest and no one responds to your shouts for help, leave the bedside in order to call the cardiac arrest team and obtain the crash trolley.

STATION 3.2: CHOKING

SCENARIO

You are on the medical wards during patients' lunch-time, and you notice that a female patient in the bay where you are starts holding her neck and cannot speak.

OBJECTIVES

- To recognise a patient who is choking
- To treat a patient who is choking

GENERAL ADVICE

- A resuscitation mannequin will be used to simulate a choking patient.
- Have a systematic approach, and take time to ensure the patient is actually choking.

RECOGNISING THE CHOKING PATIENT

- Choking most commonly occurs whilst a patient is eating.
- Classically, the choking patient will clutch their neck.
- Asking the patient if they think they are choking can be helpful. Their response will help you determine the severity of the airway obstruction.

Mild Airway Obstruction	Severe Airway Obstruction
Able to speak in words or short sentences	Unable to speak
Able to cough	May be able to nod their head in response to questions
Able to breathe	Unable to cough Unable to breathe May be unconscious

TREATING AIRWAY OBSTRUCTION

Follow the adult choking algorithm outlined in Fig. 3.12.

MILD OBSTRUCTION

1. Encourage coughing.
2. Talk to the patient and reassure them.
3. Continually reassess the patient for possible deterioration.
4. Call for assistance.

SEVERE OBSTRUCTION

1. Call for help and perform back blows.
2. Stand to the side and slightly behind the patient.
3. With one hand support the chest and lean the patient forward.
4. Give up to five back blows. These are given one at a time using the heel of your other hand in between the patient's shoulder blades (Fig. 3.13).

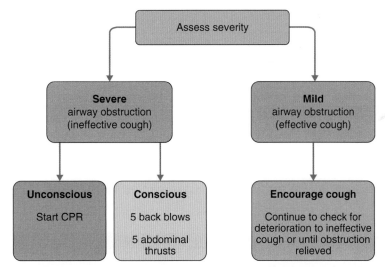

Fig. 3.12 Resuscitation Council (UK) adult choking algorithm. (Source: Reproduced by the kind permission of the Resuscitation Council (UK))

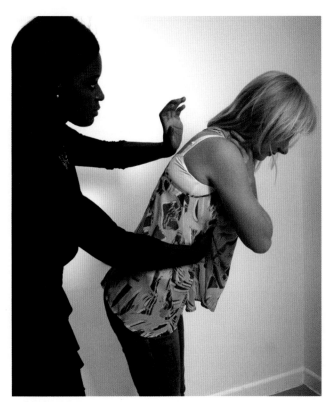

Fig. 3.13 Give the back blows quickly and firmly.

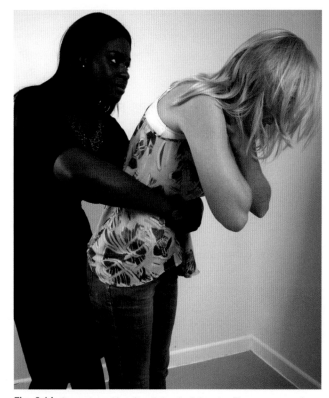

Fig. 3.14 Correct position for abdominal thrusts. Ensure you perform them in an up and inwards direction.

5. Check after each back blow to see if the obstruction has been dislodged.

If this has failed to relieve the obstruction, perform abdominal thrusts:

1. Stand behind the patient.
2. Place both your arms around their upper abdomen.
3. Lean the patient forwards as far as you can manage.
4. Form a fist with one hand (tucking your thumb in), and place it between the umbilicus and xiphoid process of the sternum.
5. Clench your fist with the other hand (Fig. 3.14).
6. Give up to five abdominal thrusts. These are given one at a time by sharply pulling upwards and inwards.

7. Check after each thrust to see if the obstruction has been dislodged.

If this has failed, then continue to alternate five back blows and five abdominal thrusts.

UNCONSCIOUS PATIENT WITH SEVERE AIRWAY OBSTRUCTION

Call for help. If the patient stops breathing, i.e. there is a respiratory arrest, call the crash team. If the patient has a pulse, ventilate at a rate of 10–12 breaths/min, while checking for pulse every minute. If a respiratory arrest is not treated promptly, it will inevitably cause a cardiac arrest.

Mark Scheme for Examiner

	0	1	2	3
Treating Mild Obstruction				
Encourages coughing				
Constantly reassesses the patient				
Treating Severe Obstruction				
Calls for help.				
Gives up to 5 back blows				
Constantly reassesses the patient				
Patient Still Obstructed				
Gives up to 5 abdominal thrusts				
Constantly reassesses the patient				
Treating an Unconscious Patient with Obstruction				
Follows procedure for ILS				
Finishing				
Ensures the patient is stable before leaving				
Documents incident in patient's notes and informs team				

0 = Not attempted
1 = Performed, with room for improvement
2 = Adequately performed
3 = Performed beyond level expected

QUESTIONS AND ANSWERS FOR CANDIDATE

What are the complications of choking?
- Aspiration pneumonia
- Lung abscess
- Gastric rupture – from abdominal thrusts
- Splenic rupture – from abdominal thrusts
- Hypoxic brain injury
- Death

What is the commonest cause of choking in children?
- Food
- Other common causes include toys and household items

How do you give back blows?
- Firmly hit the patient between the shoulder blades with the heel of your hand.

Which patients in the hospital are more likely to have an unsafe swallow?
- Patients who have had a stroke
- Patients with neurological conditions; for example, myasthenia gravis, motor neurone disease, cerebral palsy
- Patients with an obstruction in the oesophagus; for example, oesophageal cancer

How do you assess a patient's swallow at the bedside?
- Usually we ask the speech and language therapy (SALT) team to assess the patient's swallowing function.
- They may inspect the mouth, paying particular attention to the tongue, cheek, jaw, teeth and soft palate.
- They may test the gag and coughing reflex.
- They may ask the patient to swallow substances of different consistencies; for example, water, thickened liquids, puréed food, soft food and regular food.

 Tip Box

Once a patient has been successfully treated for choking, it is important to ensure that they undergo a full assessment to check the airway and for any possible complications.

 Fact Box

It is important to establish that choking is occurring, rather than an alternative diagnosis, because the management will be different. Conditions that may present similarly are myocardial infarction (MI), seizure and syncope.

STATION 3.3: SIZING AND FITTING A HARD COLLAR

SCENARIO

Mr Austin is a 28-year-old man who was involved in a road traffic accident. Please size and fit a hard cervical collar for the patient.

OBJECTIVES

- To size a hard cervical collar
- To fit a hard cervical collar

GENERAL ADVICE

- The two main types of cervical collars are hard and soft.
  - **A hard collar** is usually the first type of collar used when a patient requires cervical spine stabilisation. The hard collar is kept in place until a complete set of spinal X-rays has been taken and verified as normal.
  - **A soft collar** is used for minor injuries; for example, whiplash. It is the least limiting collar and allows for neck movement.
- Before sizing and fitting the collar, ensure the patient is supine. Explain the procedure to the patient and obtain verbal consent. Until the patient has a collar fitted, keep the cervical spine in its anatomical position, and prevent any flexion or extension.

SIZING A HARD COLLAR

1. Wash your hands.
2. Measure the patient's neck from the top of the shoulder to the bottom of the chin, using your fingers (Fig. 3.15).

3. Measure the collar from the edge of the plastic at the bottom to the sizing point or post (Fig. 3.16).

FITTING A HARD COLLAR

1. Ensure a colleague has the patient's head stabilised in alignment (Fig. 3.17).

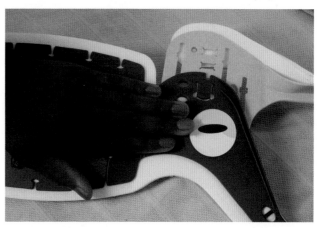

Fig. 3.16 Compare the size of the patient's neck to the collar.

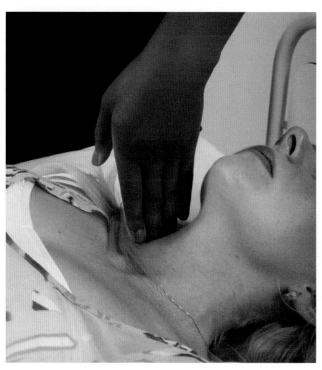

Fig. 3.15 Using your fingers is a quick and easy way to size a collar.

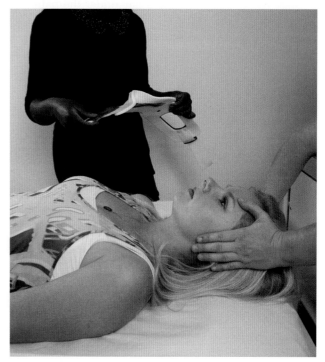

Fig. 3.17 Ensure the patient's head is stabilised.

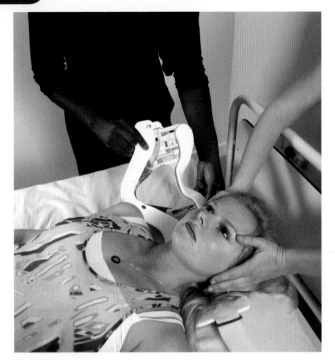

Fig. 3.18 Carefully place the collar around the patient's neck.

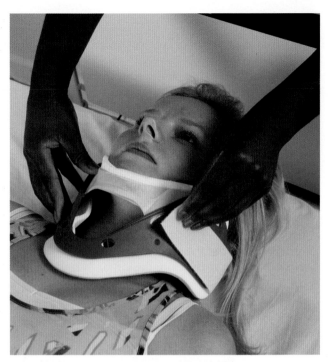

Fig. 3.19 Check that the collar fits once it is in place.

2. Slide the back half of the collar under the patient's neck (Fig. 3.18).
3. Slide the chin piece under the chin.
4. Ask your colleague to release their grip slowly.

5. Quickly fasten the pieces together using the Velcro attached to the collar (Fig. 3.19).
6. Check that the attachments are secure.
7. Check the patient's head and neck alignment.

Mark Scheme for Examiner

	0	1	2	3
Introduction and General Advice				
Introduces self, and washes hands				
Confirms patient's identity with three points of identification				
Explains procedure, identifies concerns and obtains consent (if possible)				
Ensures patient's head is being stabilised by a colleague				
Sizing a Hard Collar				
Measures patient's neck				
Chooses appropriately sized collar				
Fitting a Hard Collar				
Slides the back half of the collar under the patient's neck				
Slides in chin piece				
Asks colleague to release their grip slowly Fastens collar in place				
Checks collar is secure				
Finishing				
Orders cervical spine X-ray				

0 = Not attempted
1 = Performed, with room for improvement
2 = Adequately performed
3 = Performed beyond level expected

❓ QUESTIONS AND ANSWERS FOR CANDIDATE

What is the commonest complication of a hard collar?

- Pressure injuries are a possible complication of hard collars. Collars should be removed at least once a day to check for this. Hard collars can also be washed with soap and water.

Which patients would you want to immobilise?

- Any patient with a history of trauma with loss of consciousness, neck pain, neurological deficit or significant head injuries

Name three situations in which you would consider a cervical spine injury.

- Dangerous mechanism; for example:
  - Fall from height
  - Ejected from a vehicle
  - Severe head injury
  - Trauma to vertebral column
- Neurological symptoms suggestive of spinal cord injury
- Reduced Glasgow Coma Scale (GCS) after trauma
- Injuries above the clavicle

When can a hard collar be removed?

- A cervical collar can be removed when the following criteria are met:
  - No midline cervical spine tenderness;
  - No pain with neck movement;
  - No distracting injury;
  - No neurological deficit;
  - Not intoxicated;
  - No altered mental status; or
  - Normal computed tomography (CT) report of the cervical spine

Which views would be taken when imaging the cervical spine?

- In the absence of CT, five views of the cervical spine should be obtained:
  - Anteroposterior
  - Lateral
  - Anteroposterior oblique
  - Posteroanterior oblique
  - Odontoid

 Tip Box

Measuring a patient for a hard collar is not exact. Remember, there are only a few different sizes of collar.

 Fact Box

The Canadian cervical spine rules or NEXUS low-risk criteria can be used to determine whether imaging of the cervical spine is required.

STATION 3.4: AIRWAY MANAGEMENT

SCENARIO

In front of you lies a mannequin and a selection of airway adjuncts. Please demonstrate to the examiner: jaw-thrust, head tilt, and chin lift. How would you correctly size and insert the airway adjuncts shown in order to support the patient's airway?

OBJECTIVES

- Know how to use basic repositioning manoeuvres to maintain airway patency
- Be able to recognise a selection of airway adjuncts, and know when to use them
- Know how to size and insert such adjuncts correctly

REPOSITIONING MANOEUVRES

- **Head tilt, chin lift:** Place one hand beneath the patient's chin and the other beneath their occiput, then lift the chin, simultaneously tilting the head backwards. This is also known as the 'sniffing the morning air' position (Fig. 3.20).
- **Jaw-thrust:** From behind the patient, place the tips of the fingers from both of your hands beneath the angle of the mandible and lift. If there is any suspicion of cervical injury, a jaw-thrust should be used instead of the head tilt, chin lift method (Fig. 3.21).

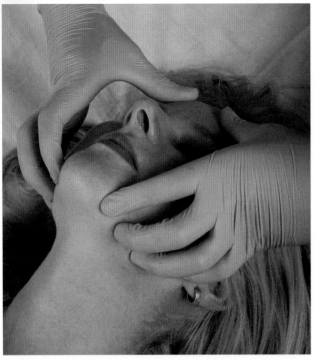

Fig. 3.20 Careful head tilt, chin lift is an important manoeuvre to perform correctly.

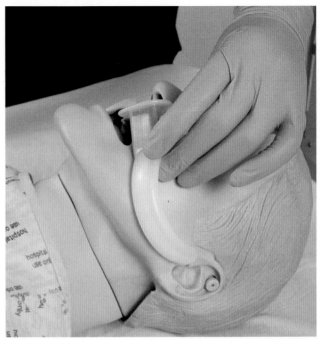

Fig. 3.22 Before using an OP airway, it must be sized correctly.

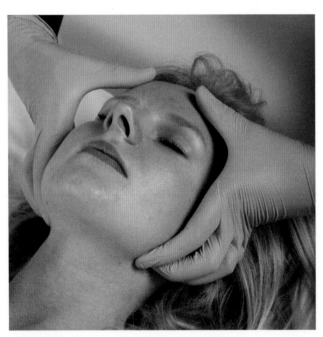

Fig. 3.21 A jaw-thrust protects the cervical spine.

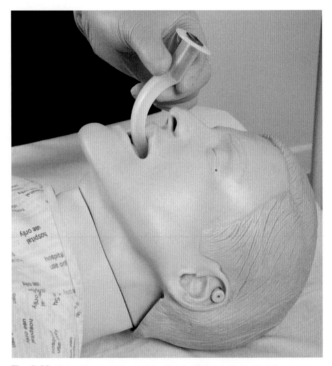

Fig. 3.23 Enter the mouth upside down. This ensures that the tongue is not pushed backwards to obstruct the airway.

ADJUNCT: OROPHARYNGEAL (OP) AIRWAY

This comprises a curved tube with bite block and flange, which are colour-coded according to size.

TO SIZE CORRECTLY

Hold the OP airway adjacent to the mannequin's jaw. A correctly sized airway will span from the incisors to the angle of the mandible (Fig. 3.22).

TO INSERT CORRECTLY

1. Holding the OP airway by the flange, insert it into the mouth upside down (with the tip pointing superiorly) (Fig. 3.23).
2. Proceed to advance the OP airway into the mouth, rotating it by 180 degrees along its long axis as you do so (Fig. 3.24).
3. Stop once the bite block rests between the teeth (Fig. 3.25).
4. Look, listen and feel for air movement to ensure patency.

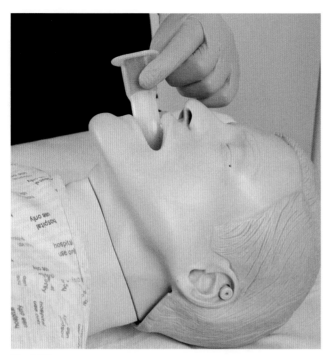

Fig. 3.24 Remember to rotate the airway whilst advancing.

ADJUNCT: NASOPHARYNGEAL AIRWAY

This comprises a flange, body and bevelled opening. Various sizes are available, as indicated by the number printed on the side of the airway.

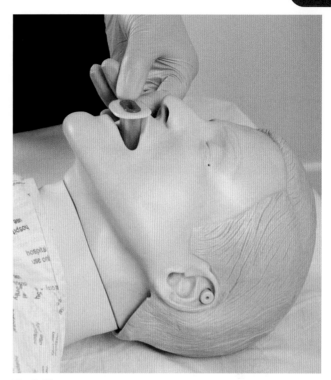

Fig. 3.25 A fully inserted OP airway.

TO SIZE CORRECTLY

Hold the nasopharyngeal airway adjacent to the mannequin's head. An 8-mm airway is usually indicated in men and a 7-mm airway for women. It is also important to adjust the size of the airway depending on the ease of passage.

TO INSERT CORRECTLY

1. Lubricate the airway adjunct to aid insertion (Fig. 3.26).
2. Introduce the bevel end into one of the nostrils and advance the airway along the floor of the nasal passage (Fig. 3.27).
3. Continue until only the flange remains at the opening of the nasal passage.

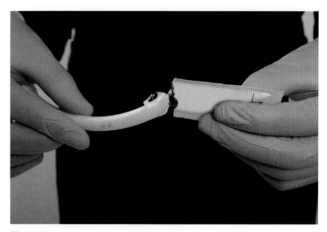

Fig. 3.26 Lubrication will assist insertion.

SUPRAGLOTTIC AIRWAY DEVICES

Laryngeal mask airway (LMA) and i-gel are airway devices that offer increased airway protection than the adjuncts mentioned above, as they are sited above the larynx. They are usually inserted in patients with a GCS <8. Supraglottic airway devices are easier to insert than ET tubes.

TO INSERT THE LMA OR I-GEL CORRECTLY
LMA

1. Remember to deflate and lubricate the cuff before insertion.

2. Insert the LMA, holding it like a pen, until you feel resistance at the back of the pharynx (Fig. 3.28).
3. Inflate the cuff using room air (Fig. 3.29).
4. Ensure the device is in situ, and that you are achieving effective ventilation, by assessing for breath sounds or chest movement.

i-gel

1. An i-gel cannot be deflated.
2. A gastric tube can be passed through it.
3. Insert the i-gel, holding it like a pen, until you feel resistance at the back of the pharynx.

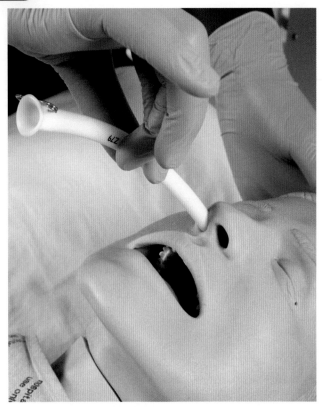

Fig. 3.27 Initially aim backwards towards the occiput, then follow the downwards curve of the airway.

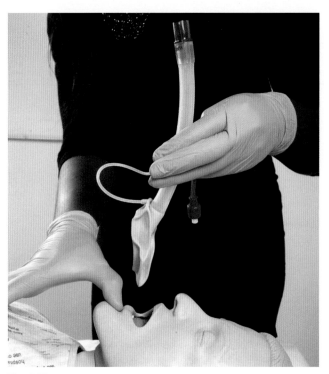

Fig. 3.28 Ensure you hold the equipment correctly.

❓ QUESTIONS AND ANSWERS FOR CANDIDATE

When should the head tilt, chin lift manoeuvre not be performed?
- Whenever there is a suspicion of possible cervical spine injury, use the jaw-thrust manoeuvre.

What is the most important contraindication to nasopharyngeal airway insertion?
- Basal skull fracture

What signs and symptoms may suggest airway obstruction?
- Signs of anaphylaxis; for example, angioedema or rash
- Sooty sputum
- Facial trauma
- Surgical emphysema
- Laboured breathing and wheeze
- Added airway noises or snoring
- Abnormal chest and abdominal wall movement
- Lack of misting of oxygen mask

Name three complications of intubation.
- Injury to teeth
- Injury to the throat or trachea
- Aspiration
- Bleeding
- Lung complications or injury

What can you do to reduce the risk of aspiration if a patient is actively vomiting or there is a significant amount of blood in the airway?

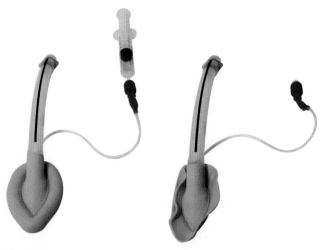

Fig. 3.29 LMA inflated, post-insertion (left) and LMA deflated, ready for insertion (right).

- Turn the patient on their side and tilt the bed/trolley head down. However, do not do this if there is suspicion of a cervical spine injury.

 Tip Box

Do not use a nasopharyngeal airway in the patient where basal skull fracture is strongly suspected. A nasopharyngeal airway could potentially enter the cranium through the disrupted skull base.

 Fact Box

Always remember to consider whether or not a patient with a decreased level of consciousness can maintain their own airway. A patient who responds only to pain (AVPU: alert, verbal, pain, unresponsive) or scores <8 on the GCS should arouse suspicion.

STATION 3.5: ADMINISTERING OXYGEN

SCENARIO

You are a junior doctor working in the emergency department when Mr Hill, a 62-year-old man, presents acutely short of breath. A nurse performs a set of basic observations, which reveal his oxygen saturations to be 85%. You decide this patient requires supplementary oxygen therapy. Discuss what methods for delivering oxygen are available and which may be most appropriate in this situation.

OBJECTIVES

- Be aware of the various methods available for delivering supplementary oxygen
- Be able to determine which method is most appropriate for a given scenario

GENERAL ADVICE

- There are several ways in which supplementary oxygen can be delivered.
- Titrate the oxygen you administer according to the patient's oxygen saturations.
- As with medications, oxygen should be prescribed on a drug chart.

NASAL CANNULAE – THE STABLE PATIENT

- Nasal cannulae consist of a length of oxygen tubing with two nasal prongs and are looped over the ears and beneath the chin (Fig. 3.30).
- They are typically preferred by the patient for comfort.
- Beware:
  - The amount of oxygen delivered is variable and imprecise.

Mark Scheme for Examiner

	0	1	2	3
General				
Washes hands				
Puts on non-sterile gloves				
Airway Manoeuvres				
Performs head tilt, chin lift				
Performs jaw-thrusts correctly				
Airway Adjuncts				
Correctly identifies OP airway				
Chooses appropriately sized OP for mannequin				
Uses correct insertion technique				
Correctly identifies nasopharyngeal airway				
Chooses appropriate size for mannequin				
Uses correct insertion technique				
Advanced Airway (LMA/igel)				
Correctly identifies LMA/igel				
Prepares LMA/igel for insertion				
Uses correct insertion technique				
Checks positioning by assessing breath sounds and/or chest wall movements				
General Points				
Talks clearly to the examiner throughout the station				
Remains calm and works methodically				

0 = Not attempted
1 = Performed, with room for improvement
2 = Adequately performed
3 = Performed beyond level expected

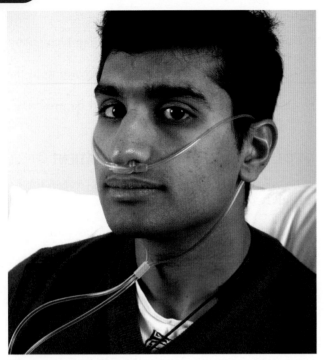

Fig. 3.30 Nasal cannulae in situ.

- Nasal soreness or epistaxis may arise from higher flow rates or prolonged use.
- Achievable flow rate: 1–4 L/min.
- Achievable FiO_2: 24%–40%.

SIMPLE MASK — THE ACUTELY ILL PATIENT

- A transparent face mask with an oxygen tubing connector and elasticity strap
- Less comfortable than the nasal cannulae (Fig. 3.31)
- Beware:
  - It must be used with follow rate of 5–10 L/min (if less than 5 L is used, excessive levels of CO_2 can accumulate within the mask).
  - These masks should be avoided in patients at risk of type 2 respiratory failure.
  - Achievable flow rate: 5–10 L/min.
  - Achievable FiO_2: 40%–60%.

Due to long-standing hypercapnia, patients in type 2 respiratory failure may have a hypoxia-driven respiratory centre. Care should be taken in administering oxygen to these patients as administering too much will cause them to become apnoeic. Start with a Venturi face mask FiO_2 24%–28% and aim for target saturations of 88%–92%. Make sure that the nursing staff are aware of this target range.

VENTURI MASK — THE ACUTELY ILL PATIENT WHO MAY DEVELOP TYPE 2 RESPIRATORY FAILURE (FOR EXAMPLE, KNOWN CHRONIC OBSTRUCTIVE PULMONARY DISEASE (COPD))

- Similar in appearance to the simple face mask but with the addition of a specially designed (and

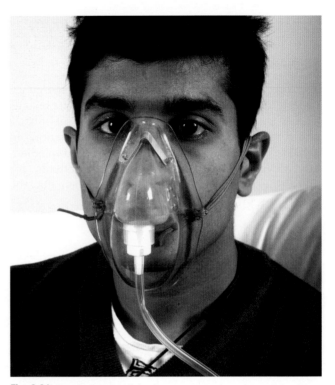

Fig. 3.31 Simple face mask in situ.

colour-coded) adapter allowing a precise FiO_2 to be administered
- For use when it is crucially important to deliver a fixed and specific FiO_2 (i.e. in type 2 respiratory failure) (Fig. 3.32)
- Beware:
  - You must ensure that you select the correct adapter for your patient, and review their oxygen saturations regularly.
  - Achievable flow rate: dependent on the colour-coded adapter (see below).
  - Achievable FiO_2: 24%–60%.

Possible FiO_2 that may be achieved using the Venturi face mask	
60% (12 L/min)	Green
40% (10 L/min)	Red
35% (8 L/min)	Yellow
28% (4 L/min)	White
24% (2 L/min)	Blue

NON-REBREATHER MASK — THE CRITICALLY ILL PATIENT

- Non-rebreather masks comprise a face mask plus reservoir bag.
- By using a high-flow rate, a reservoir bag can deliver a high FiO_2 (Fig. 3.33).
- The reservoir bag needs to be filled with air before use.
- Beware:

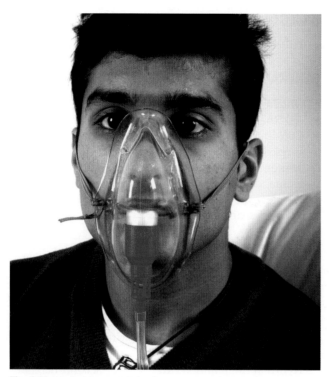

Fig. 3.32 Venturi face mask in situ.

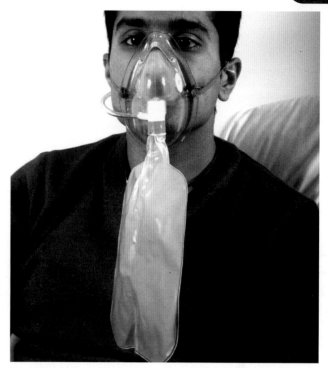

Fig. 3.33 Non-rebreather mask in situ.

- The use of a non-rebreather mask is not recommended in patients who require precisely controlled O_2 delivery.
- It is often used in emergency or trauma situations.
- Achievable flow rate: 10–15 L/min.
- Achievable FiO_2: 60%–90%.

FiO_2

This is the fraction or percentage of oxygen in the space being measured. Natural air contains 21% oxygen, which correlates to an FiO_2 of 0.21.

PaO_2

This is the partial pressure of oxygen gas, dissolved in the blood. It can only be measured by performing an arterial blood gas analysis.

Respiratory Failure

Type 1	Type 2
Failure to oxygenate	Failure to oxygenate
PaO_2 <8 kPa	PaO_2 <8 kPa
$PaCO_2$ = normal or low	$PaCO_2$ >6 kPa

❓ QUESTIONS AND ANSWERS FOR CANDIDATE

What would be the most appropriate method for use in the case of Mr Hill?
- A non-rebreather face mask with high-flow oxygen (10–15 L/min), provided he has no underlying lung pathology contraindicating high-flow oxygen

Why is high-flow oxygen potentially problematic in patients with type 2 respiratory failure?

- Due to long-standing hypercapnia, these patients may have a hypoxia-driven respiratory centre. High-flow oxygen could suppress this drive, resulting in apnoea.

Name three possible indications for bilevel positive airway pressure (BiPAP).
- Hypercapnic respiratory failure, i.e. type 2 respiratory failure
- Postoperative or posttraumatic respiratory failure
- COPD with respiratory acidosis
- Weaning from tracheal intubation
- Acute asthma
- Cardiogenic pulmonary oedema
- Obstructive sleep apnoea

What are some contraindications to non-invasive ventilation (NIV)?
- Upper-airway obstruction
- Inability to protect the airway; for example, impaired consciousness
- Untreated pneumothorax
- Cardiac or respiratory arrest
- Haemodynamically unstable
- Base-of-skull facture
- Intractable vomiting
- Facial trauma or injury

Describe the difference between BiPAP and continuous positive airway pressure (CPAP) ventilation.
- BiPAP is a form of NIV, which delivers differing air pressure depending on inspiration and expiration. Inspiratory positive airway pressure is usually greater than the expiratory positive airway pressure, typically used in type 2 respiratory failure.
- CPAP provides a constant, fixed positive pressure through inspiration and expiration. It is not a form

of ventilation, but it supplies a higher degree of inspired oxygen, typically used in type 1 respiratory failure.

 Tip Box

An arterial blood gas provides the PaO_2, which can be helpful both in terms of planning how to deliver oxygen and to determine how much to provide. Therefore, arterial blood gas should *always* be considered when you are asked to review a patient who is experiencing breathing difficulties.

 Fact Box

The *flow rate* refers to the value you should adjust the oxygen wall outlet to; for example, 10 L/min or 5 L/min.

STATION 3.6: INTRAVENOUS CANNULATION

SCENARIO

Mrs Jones has been diagnosed with small-bowel obstruction. She requires cannulation so that IV fluids can be administered. Please obtain consent for this and then, on the mannequin provided, demonstrate how to insert an IV cannula.

OBJECTIVES

- To learn correct technique for cannula insertion

GENERAL ADVICE

- Obtain consent.
- Ask the patient if they have an arm preference.
- Consider if there are any predisposing medical or surgical conditions that would not allow a specific arm or blood vessel to be used; for example, a renal fistula, cellulitis or mastectomy.
- Check if the patient has any allergies; for example, to chlorhexidine.

EQUIPMENT CHECKLIST

(Remember to check expiry dates on all equipment) (Fig. 3.34).)
- Skin-cleansing solution; for example, ChloraPrep
- 21-gauge needle (though, for drawing up medications, in *all* cases a blunt draw-up needle is preferred if available)
- 10-mL syringe and syringe cap (or second needle if syringe cap is not available)
- 10-mL 0.9% saline ampoule for flush
- Sterile adhesive dressing

Mark Scheme for Examiner

	0	1	2	3
Nasal Cannulae				
Correctly identifies equipment				
Describes correct method of application				
States that these are for use in a stable patient				
States correct achievable flow rates (1–4 L/min) and FiO_2 (24%–40%)				
Simple Face Mask				
Correctly identifies equipment				
Describes correct method of application				
States that this is for use in an acutely ill patient				
States correct achievable flow rates (5–10 L/min) and FiO_2 (40%–60%)				
Venturi Mask				
Correctly identifies equipment				
Describes correct method of application				
States that this is for use in an acutely ill patient when a precise FiO_2 is required				
Mentions type 2 respiratory failure or COPD as appropriate indications				
States that there are a range of colour-coded adapters to be used with various flow rates in order to achieve different FiO_2 values				
Non-Rebreathe Mask				
Correctly identifies equipment				
Describes correct method of application and the need to fill reservoir bag				
States that this is for use in a critically ill patient				
States correct achievable flow rates (10–15 L/min) and FiO_2 (60%–90%)				
General Points				
Talks clearly to the examiner throughout the station				

0 = Not attempted
1 = Performed, with room for improvement
2 = Adequately performed
3 = Performed beyond level expected

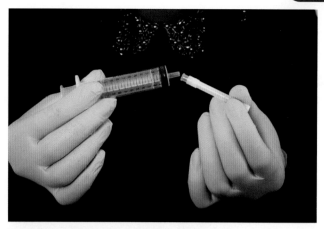
Fig. 3.35 Prepare your needle and syringe.

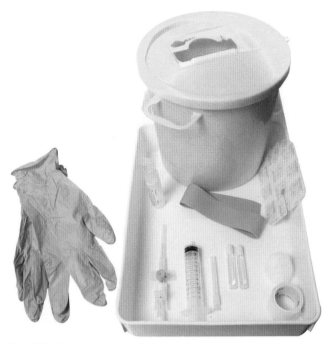
Fig. 3.34 Equipment required for cannulation.

- Cannula
- Disposable tourniquet
- Cotton wool
- Two pairs of non-sterile gloves
- Tape (if you fail to site the cannula you will need to tape some cotton wool over the puncture site)
- Tray (as with phlebotomy)
- Sharps bin: the sharps bin should always be taken to the point of care
- Single-use disposable apron

Note: Skin-cleansing methods and methods of capping will vary depending on local policy. In addition, local policy may use alternative methods to cap. Any tubing that is attached, such as a bioconnector or a line, needs to be flushed first with 0.9% saline to avoid injecting air and risking an air embolus.

EXPLAINING IV CANNULATION TO THE PATIENT

1. A cannula is a small plastic tube that remains in your vein, allowing you to receive fluid and medication.
2. It is inserted using a needle, a bit like having a blood test. You will feel a sharp scratch but the needle is removed once the plastic tube is in place.
3. It is held in place with a sticky dressing.
4. The cannula will be changed every 3 days if you need it for a longer period of time.
5. It may take a few attempts to ensure the plastic tube is in the correct place.

PERFORMING THE PROCEDURE

PREPARING THE FLUSH

1. Clean hands and put on non-sterile gloves.

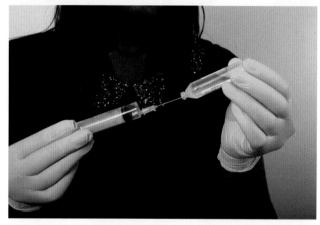
Fig. 3.36 Draw up the saline flush.

2. Attach the 21-gauge needle to the 10-mL syringe (leave the sheath on for now) (Fig. 3.35).
3. Double check that you have selected 0.9% saline, that it is in date and that the packaging is clean and intact — many IV medications appear in near-identical ampoules.
4. Remove the top from the 0.9% saline and draw 10 mL up into your syringe using a 21-gauge needle (Fig. 3.36).
5. Expel any air from the syringe by tapping it or advancing the plunger (Fig. 3.37).
6. Discard the needle in the sharps bin and attach the syringe to the second needle for storage (or if available, a sterilised cap for the syringe tip).
7. Place the flush into the equipment tray alongside the other cannulation equipment.

INSERTING THE CANNULA

1. Remove the cannula from its packaging and open the sterile dressing pack.
2. Position the patient's arm comfortably.
3. Place the tourniquet approximately 7–10 cm proximal to the site of inserting (Fig. 3.38).
4. Select vein, then loosen the tourniquet.

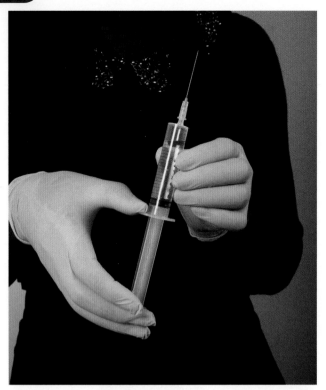

Fig. 3.37 Expel any air present.

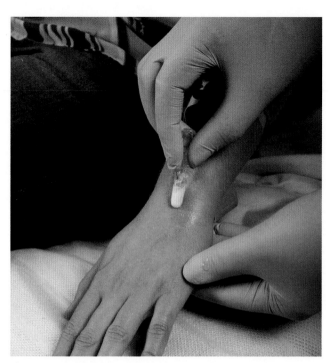

Fig. 3.39 Carefully clean cannula insertion site.

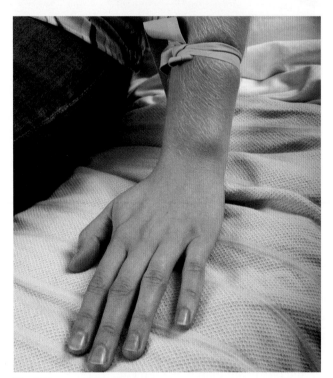

Fig. 3.38 Ensure tourniquet is out of the sterile field.

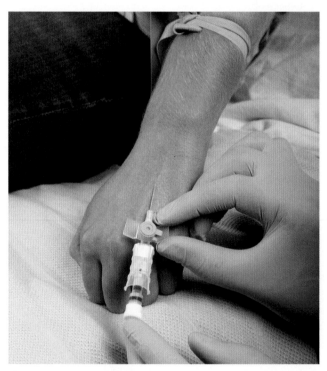

Fig. 3.40 Enter the skin using NTT.

5. Wash hands, put on new non-sterile gloves and apron.
6. Clean the site using the skin-cleansing solution — clean for 30 s and leave to air dry (Fig. 3.39).
7. Retighten the tourniquet.
8. Tether the vein that you have selected beneath the insertion site and insert the cannula at approximately 15 degrees using non-touch technique (NTT), while warning the patient of a 'sharp scratch' (Fig. 3.40).
9. Advance the cannula until flashback is obtained. Do not repalpate the aseptic area of the skin at any time during the procedure.
10. Once flashback has been seen, advance the cannula slightly further (1—2 mm). This ensures the

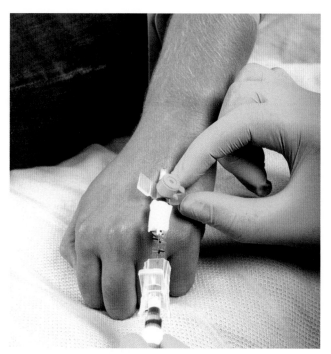

Fig. 3.41 Cannula is fully inserted.

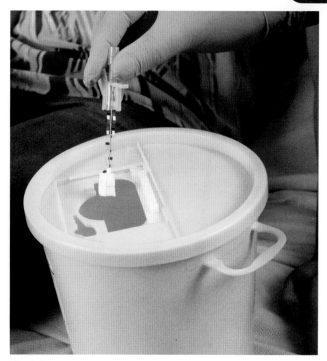

Fig. 3.43 Ensure you have a sharps bin nearby.

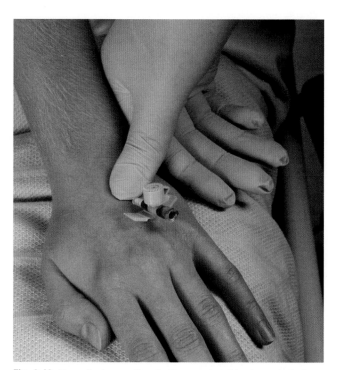

Fig. 3.42 Press firmly over the plastic cannula tubing to occlude it.

cannula tubing is within the vein before you advance it forward, over and off the needle.

11. Hold the needle still and advance the cannula over it, all the way into the vein. No part of the cannula tubing must be seen at the point of entry (Fig. 3.41).
12. Release the tourniquet.
13. Occlude the vein and cannula with firm pressure (Fig. 3.42), and then gently remove the needle.

14. Dispose of the needle straight into the sharps bin (Fig. 3.43).
15. Depending on Trust policy, attach a cap, bung or IV extension set (which requires separate preparation) on the end of the cannula.
16. Wipe away any blood that may have leaked around the cannula with cotton wool.
17. Apply sterile adhesive dressing (Fig. 3.44).
18. Write the date and time on the cannula dressing label.

FLUSHING THE CANNULA

1. Flip open the coloured cap of the cannula (note, however, if an IV extension set is applied, you would flush the cannula through this, not the coloured cap).
2. Remove the needle or sterilised cap from the saline flush syringe and attach the flush to the cannula.
3. Slowly flush the cannula (1 mL at a time) with 5–10 mL of 0.9% saline, checking that the fluid does not leak into the surrounding tissues, causing swelling (Fig. 3.45).
4. Explain to the patient that they might feel coldness running up their arm as you are flushing the cannula.
5. When finished, remove the syringe and recap the cannula.
6. Dispose of the syringe in a sharps bin.

FINISHING

1. Decontaminate tray as per local policy.
2. Dispose of equipment in a clinical waste bin.
3. Remove gloves.

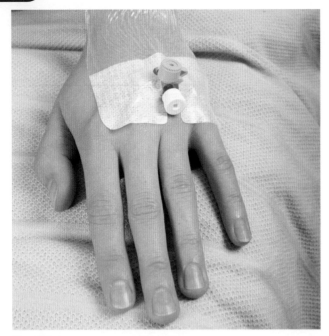

Fig. 3.44 Secure the cannula in place.

4. Wash hands.
5. Complete a cannula insertion record, and place in notes.
6. Explain to the patient that if they have any other concerns, they should speak to a member of staff.

DOCUMENT THE PROCEDURE

Document under the following headings:
- IV cannulation performed
- Date, time and place
- Indications for the procedure
- Patient consent
- Site used
- Number of attempts
- Complications

❓ QUESTIONS AND ANSWERS FOR CANDIDATE

What cannula would you use for a blood transfusion?
- If it was a scheduled blood transfusion, a pink (20G) cannula would be sufficient, but a green cannula (22G) is recommended. If it was an emergency, a larger cannula would be preferred.

Name two complications of IV cannulation.
- Phlebitis
- Entry site infection
- Blood stream infection
- Extravasation

When might you remove a cannula?
- When venous access is no longer required
- After a prolonged period of time in situ (this varies depending on local Trust policy, but usually after 72–96 h)

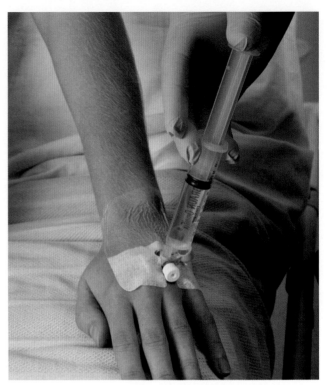

Fig. 3.45 Always flush the cannula after insertion.

- When the cannula is no longer working
- If there are complications; for example, pain, redness, swelling, other signs of infection

What factor is the most critical determinant of flow rate through a cannula?
- The main limiting factor of flow rate through a cannula is the lumen diameter and length of the cannula.
- Other factors include the viscosity of the fluid and the pressure of infusion.

In an emergency, if you cannot gain IV access, what other routes are acceptable for drug delivery?
- Intraosseous

💡 Tip Box
Patient comfort is important in considering where to place the cannula, particularly in non-emergency situations. Put it in the left arm if they are right-handed, use a small cannula if that is all that might be needed. Remember that although the antecubital fossa is tempting, placing a cannula here makes it more difficult to move the arm.

Fact Box
Cannulae are sized by gauge (the smaller the number, the bigger the size), all with corresponding colours. Bigger cannulae can achieve higher flow rates. For administering IV medication and IV maintenance fluids, smaller cannulae (pink/blue) are fine. In an emergency, a large cannula is preferred (green or bigger) since this permits more rapid administration of medications and fluids.

STATION 3.7: SETTING UP A GIVING SET

SCENARIO

Mrs Jones has been diagnosed with small-bowel obstruction. She has a cannula in situ and now requires maintenance fluid. Please obtain consent for this and then, on the cannulated mannequin provided, demonstrate how to assemble a giving set and commence IV fluid therapy.

OBJECTIVES

- To learn how to set up a giving set

GENERAL ADVICE

- Check whether the patient has any concerns or questions and obtain consent.
- Check if the patient has any allergies.
- There are two types of giving sets, one for blood transfusions and another for general use.

EQUIPMENT CHECKLIST

(Remember to check the expiry dates on all equipment (Fig. 3.46).)
- IV fluid; for example, 1 L 0.9% saline
- Gravity administration set ('giving set')
- Drip stand
- Skin-cleansing solution; for example, ChloraPrep
- 10-mL syringe
- Sterile gauze
- Tray
- Sharps bin: the sharps bin should always be taken to the point of care
- Two pairs of non-sterile gloves

Note: Skin-cleansing solutions and method will vary depending on local policy.

SETTING UP THE GIVING SET

PREPARATION

1. Wash hands, and put on non-sterile gloves.
2. Check the bag of fluid with the examiner:
   - Is it the same fluid and quantity as prescribed on the fluid chart?
   - Are any additives required; for example, potassium or magnesium?
   - Is it in date?
   - Check that there is no sediment floating in the fluid bag.
   - Check that the bag has not leaked into the packaging.
3. Remove the bag of fluid from its outer packaging, and hang it on the drip stand.
4. Remove the giving set from the bag and roll the flow control wheel down to the 'off' position. The 'off' position is where the tube is clamped, ensuring that the fluid does not run through the line onto the floor (Fig. 3.47).
5. Remove the cap from the fluid bag by twisting it, and remove the protective cover from the trocar of the giving set. The trocar is a sharp hollow cylinder that pierces the fluid bag to provide a connection between the fluid and the giving set (take care not to touch either ends in order to maintain an aseptic technique) (Fig. 3.48).
6. Insert the trocar end of the giving set into the bag of fluid (push hard and twist) (Fig. 3.49).
7. Squeeze the chamber at the top of the giving set until it is filled halfway with fluid (Fig. 3.50).
8. Slowly open the flow control wheel of the giving set so that fluid flows down the line — do this bit by bit until the line is full of fluid and no air bubbles can be seen. If the line is full of bubbles, the process needs to be started again with new sterile equipment.
9. Reset the flow control wheel to the closed position.
10. Hang the bag on the drip stand. You are now ready to connect the giving set to the cannula.
11. Remove gloves.

CONNECTING THE GIVING SET TO THE CANNULA

1. Before going to the patient's bedside, draw up a saline flush (as explained in station 3.6) and place this on the equipment tray.
2. Wash hands, and put on non-sterile gloves.
3. Check patient identification.
4. Check the cannula (When was it inserted? Are there any signs of localised infection?).
5. Flush the cannula via the coloured cap with the saline (clean cannula entry site first with chlorhexidine wipe).
6. Place the gauze beneath the end of the cannula.
7. Depending on your Trust policy, there are different techniques for connecting a giving set. If there is a cannula cap, it must be swiftly removed, wiped with a chlorhexidine wipe and the giving set connected. If your Trust has a connector, this can be cleaned with a chlorhexidine wipe for 30 s and then allow 30 s for it to dry. After this, the giving set is connected (Fig. 3.51).

Mark Scheme for Examiner

	0	1	2	3
Introduction and General Advice				
Introduces self, and washes hands				
Confirms patient's identity with three points of identification				
Explains procedure, identifies concerns and obtains consent				
Checks for allergies and needle phobia, and any contraindications to use of left or right arm				
Preparation				
Obtains equipment and checks expiry dates				
Washes hands and puts on non-sterile gloves				
Assembles equipment				
Preparation of IV Flush				
Draws up saline flush using NTT				
Safely stows syringe in tray				
Cannulation				
Positions arm appropriately				
Applies disposable tourniquet, selects vein, loosening tourniquet				
Washes hands				
Puts on non-sterile gloves and single-use apron				
Cleans puncture site (30 s) and allows to air dry				
Reapplies tourniquet				
Uses appropriate insertion technique				
Removes tourniquet				
Removes needle (whilst occluding vein) and immediately disposes of sharp safely				
Attaches cap and cleans any leakage of blood				
Applies dressing with date and time				
Flushing the Cannula				
Opens coloured cap of cannula and attaches preprepared flush				
Flushes cannula 1 mL at a time				
Disposes of syringe				
Finishing				
Disposes of equipment				
Removes gloves and apron				
Washes hands				
Documents insertion				
Explains to patient to be wary of signs of infection				
General Points				
Talks to the patient throughout the procedure				
Avoids patient contamination (i.e. NTT)				

0 = Not attempted
1 = Performed, with room for improvement
2 = Adequately performed
3 = Performed beyond level expected

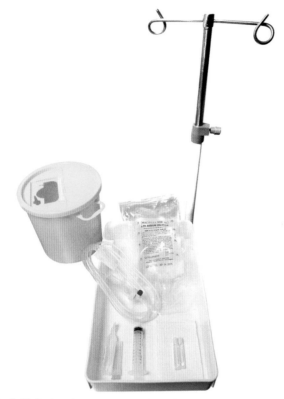

Fig. 3.46 Gather the equipment needed.

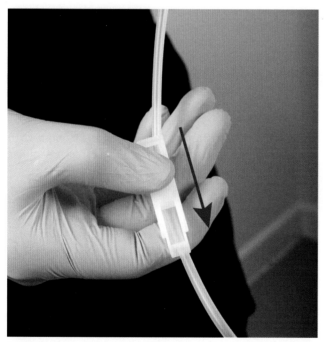

Fig. 3.47 Always turn the control wheel to the 'off' position before starting.

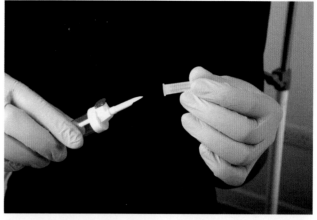

Fig. 3.48 Expose the trocar.

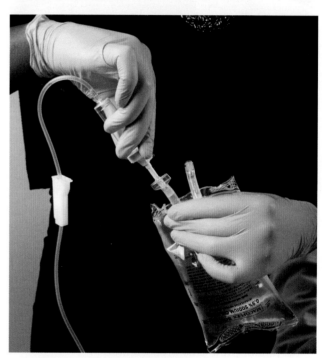

Fig. 3.49 Push and twist to insert the trocar.

DOCUMENT THE PROCEDURE

Document under the following headings:
- Giving set set up
- Date, time and place
- Indications for the giving set
- Patient consent
- Type, quantity and rate of fluid given
- Complications

❓ QUESTIONS AND ANSWERS FOR CANDIDATE

In an emergency scenario how could you maximise the rate at which you administer IV fluid?
- Insert the largest cannula size possible
- Increase drip stand height
- Squeeze fluid bag or apply pressurised cuff

FINISHING

- Dispose of equipment.
- Clean the tray.
- Dispose of gloves and wash your hands.
- Document the procedure.

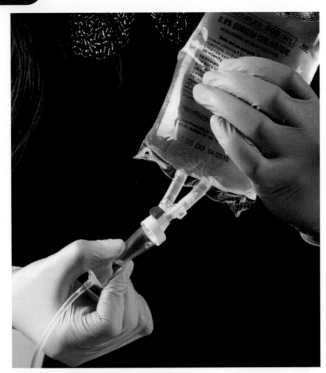

Fig. 3.50 Prepare the chamber by squeezing it.

- Insert a second cannula

What is a fluid challenge and how would you administer one?
- A fluid bolus is 500 mL of crystalloid, to be administered over less than 15 min.

What indicators may suggest that a patient requires fluid resuscitation?
- Systolic blood pressure (BP) <100 mmHg
- Heart rate >90 beats/min
- Capillary refill time (CRT) >2 s
- Cold peripheries
- Respiratory rate >20 breaths/min
- National Early Warning Score (NEWS) ≥ 5.

How would you assess the rate at which to give fluid in a dehydrated patient?

- Assess whether the patient requires fluid for maintenance, resuscitation or redistribution and replacement.

What signs and symptoms may suggest ongoing abnormal fluid or electrolyte losses?
- Vomiting and nasogastric tube loss
- Biliary drainage loss
- High-/low-volume ileal stoma loss
- Diarrhoea/excess colostomy loss
- Ongoing blood loss
- Sweatiness
- Fever
- Dehydration

💡 **Tip Box**

When you are on the wards, shadow the nurses for a bit and ask them to observe you while you put up a giving set. This allows you to get the practice and obtain useful feedback.

🐘 **Fact Box**

Broadly speaking, there are two key groups of patients requiring IV fluid:
- **Maintenance** – Patients with an insufficient oral intake
- **Resuscitation** – Patients who are hypovolaemic

STATION 3.8: BLOOD TRANSFUSION

SCENARIO

Mrs Patel is a 72-year-old woman who has been admitted to hospital with lethargy, drowsiness and shortness of breath. On examination, she has pale conjunctivae and tachypnoea. Her blood tests have come back demonstrating a normocytic anaemia with a haemoglobin (Hb) of 65 g/L. Please discuss blood transfusion with the examiner.

OBJECTIVES

- Understanding the indications, procedure and complications of blood transfusion

📖 **Mark Scheme for Examiner**

	0	1	2	3
Introduction and General Advice				
Introduces self, and washes hands				
Confirms patient's identity with three points of identification				
Explains procedure, identifies concerns and obtains consent.				
Checks for allergies, checks cannula (insertion date, infection signs), checks fluid prescription				

Continued

Mark Scheme for Examiner—cont'd

	0	1	2	3
Preparation				
Obtains equipment and checks expiry dates				
Washes hands, and puts on non-sterile gloves				
Examines fluid bag				
Removes the giving set from the bag and closes the flow control wheel				
Removes cap from the fluid bag and hangs it on the drip stand				
Inserts the trocar of the giving set into the bag of fluid				
Squeezes the chamber at the top of the giving set until it is filled halfway with fluid				
Opens flow control wheel slowly, then closes it when line is full of fluid				
Ensures IV line is free of air bubbles				
Preparation of IV Flush				
Draws up saline flush using NTT				
Safely stows syringe in tray				
Connecting the Giving Set				
Washes hands, and puts on non-sterile gloves				
Cleans end of cannula				
Uses appropriate connection technique				
Calculating the Drip Rate				
Rechecks fluid prescription (for duration of fluid therapy)				
Sets flow wheel correctly				
Finishing				
Disposes of equipment				
Removes gloves and apron				
Washes hands				
Provides appropriate documentation				
General Points				
Talks to the patient throughout the procedure				
Avoids patient contamination (i.e. NTT)				

0 = Not attempted
1 = Performed, with room for improvement
2 = Adequately performed
3 = Performed beyond level expected

GENERAL ADVICE

- Obtain consent.
- Each Trust will have a policy for the procedure of administration of blood products. Ensure that you are familiar with these before you start working.
- There is no standardised 'trigger' for transfusion.
- The decision to transfuse should be taken after considering the laboratory results, the clinical assessment of the patient as well as the risks and benefits of transfusion.
- If possible, the decision to transfuse should always be discussed with the patient.
- The reason for transfusion must be documented in the patient's notes.

EQUIPMENT CHECKLIST

(Remember to check expiry dates on all equipment.)
- Tray: Either single-use, disposable sterilised tray, or a decontaminated plastic tray that is cleaned pre-/post-procedure

- Two pairs of non-sterile gloves and single-use apron
- Skin-cleansing solution
- Prescribed blood products
- Prescribed 10 mL 0.9% saline to flush
- Blood giving set
- 10-mL syringe
- 21-gauge needle
- Sharps bin

ORDERING BLOOD PRODUCTS

There is a strict process in most Trusts with regard to ordering blood products. Most require the order form to be handwritten and signed by both the healthcare professional who ordered the blood and the person who took the blood. If there is any discrepancy between the order form and the blood sample, the order will not be processed.

TESTS TO ORDER

- **Group and save** – The blood bank analyses the sample ABO blood group, Rhesus (Rh) (D) and

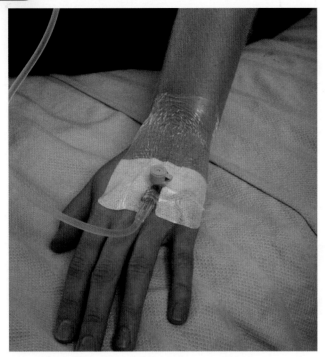

Fig. 3.51 Correctly attach the giving set to the cannula.

common red cell antibodies. This result is then stored on the hospital system.

- **Routine crossmatch** — The blood bank analyses the samples as for any antibodies against compatible blood that is stored in the hospital. This takes approximately 40 min.
- **Emergency crossmatch** — The blood bank analyses the sample's ABO blood group only. This takes approximately 10 min.

Note: Group O negative blood is kept in emergency fridges if there is not time to wait for an emergency crossmatch.

Blood Products to Order

Blood Product	Indications	Shelf-Life
Packed red cells	Acute blood loss Perioperative transfusion Symptomatic anaemia	35 days
Platelets	Active bleeding caused by platelet dysfunction	5 days
Fresh frozen plasma (FFP)	Replacing coagulation factor deficiency Disseminated intra-vascular coagulation (DIC) Massive blood transfusion Warfarin reversal (if major bleeding or emergency surgery)	1–2 years
Cryoprecipitate	Liver disease with abnormal bleeding DIC Massive blood transfusion	1–2 years

CHECKS AND PREPARATION

1. Check that the patient has given consent.
2. Wash hands and put on gloves.
3. Compare the type of blood you have received from the lab with the order form.
4. Compare the ABO blood group and Rh (D) reports, ensuring they are the same.
5. Assess the blood product you have been supplied with, checking for any abnormal colouring, gas bubbles, tampering and expiry date.
6. Confirm the patient's identity by checking the identification wristband, and asking the patient to state:
   - Full name
   - Date of birth
   - Address and postcode
   Confirm with another qualified member of staff (this is stated in some Trust policies).
7. Check that the blood donor number and the patient's number are accurate.
8. Document a full set of observations, including:
   - Respiratory rate
   - Heart rate
   - Temperature
   - BP
   - SaO_2
9. Check that the patient has a patent IV cannula in situ that has been in situ for less than 72 h.
10. Check that the cannula site has no sign of infection.
11. Collect the equipment you require, and assemble your 0.9% saline flush in a 10-mL syringe.
12. Wash hands, and don non-sterile gloves and apron.
13. Prepare the blood product using a blood giving set (as in station 3.7).

GIVING BLOOD PRODUCTS

1. Clean the coloured port of the cannula using skin-cleansing solution for 30 s and allow to dry for 30 s.
2. Check that the cannula is patent by flushing 5 mL of 0.9% saline through the coloured port of the cannula.
3. Once you are sure that the cannula is correctly in place, attach the blood transfusion giving set and start the transfusion (Fig. 3.52).
4. Wash hands and remove gloves.
5. Remain with the patient for at least 15–30 min, depending on Trust guidelines.

DOCUMENTING THE PROCEDURE

Document under the following headings:
- Date and time transfusion started
- Date and time transfusion finished
- Reason for transfusion
- Patient consent
- Type of blood product
- Number of units transfused
- Unit and batch numbers
- Outcome of transfusion
- Adverse reactions (if any) (Table 3.1)

1 unit of packed red cells will increase the Hb by approximately 10 g/L.

When do you decide to transfuse?

- This depends on the individual situation of the patient you are caring for. If you are unsure it is best to ask for advice. As a general rule, guidelines tend to recommend transfusing when a patient's Hb falls below 70–80 g/L. However, if a patient has comorbidities; for example, ischaemic heart disease, this threshold may be increased to 100 g/L. Lower transfusion thresholds are also considered in patients symptomatic of anaemia.

When would you consider giving a blood transfusion at night?

- Most trusts recommend transfusing a patient during the day as there are more staff present on the wards, and it is safer for the patient as these patients require regular observations during and after transfusion. There are specific areas in the hospital and certain situations when a transfusion will be given overnight; for example, in the Intensive Treatment Unit, Accident and Emergency and the medical or surgical assessment units. However, blood transfusions can be given at any time in an emergency.

Over what length of time should a unit of red cell concentrate be given under non-emergency circumstances?

- Over 2–4 h

Name three causes of normocytic anaemia.

- Anaemia of chronic disease; for example, renal failure, hypothyroidism, polymyalgia rheumatica
- Marrow failure (aplastic anaemia, pure red cell aplasia)
- Leukaemia

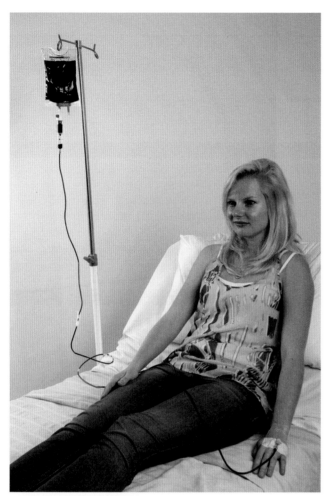

Fig. 3.52 Administer the blood product through a cannula.

- Repeat and document the patient's general observations every 5–10 min as recommended by your Trust guidelines

QUESTIONS AND ANSWERS FOR CANDIDATE

How do you know how many units to transfuse?

- This depends on the individual situation of the patient you are caring for. If you are unsure, it is best to ask the advice of a senior doctor on your team, or the duty haematologist. As a general rule,

> **Tip Box**
>
> There are numerous transfusion-related complications, some of which are highlighted in Table 3.1. An acute reaction is defined as occurring within 24 h of the transfusion being given, whilst a delayed reaction is defined as one starting after 24 h.

Table **3.1**   **Adverse reactions to blood transfusions**

Acute	
Acute haemolysis	Usually presents with: pyrexia, pain, tachycardia, hypotension and agitation
Anaphylaxis	Usually presents with: wheeze, flushing, tachypnoea, tachycardia and hypotension
Febrile non-haemolytic transfusion reaction	Usually presents with: isolated pyrexia
Transfusion-related circulatory overload	Usually presents with: hypertension, tachypnoea and tachycardia
Delayed	
Viral infection	These include: hepatitis B and hepatitis C
Delayed haemolytic reaction	As for acute haemolysis

📖 Mark Scheme for Examiner

	0	1	2	3
Introduction and General Advice				
Introduces self, and washes hands				
Confirms patient's identity with three points of identification, and confirms with another staff member				
Explains procedure, identifies concerns and obtains consent				
Preparation				
Obtains equipment, checks expiry dates, washes hands, dons gloves				
Assembles equipment				
Checks prescription				
Checks blood product, and confirms with another staff member				
Documents full set of patient observations				
Checks cannula site				
Washes hands, dons non-sterile gloves and apron				
Giving Blood Product				
Cleans cannula port and draws up saline flush				
Checks cannula patency				
Sets up blood transfusion giving set				
Starts transfusion				
Washes hands, removes gloves and apron				
Remains with patient				
Repeats and documents observations				
Disposes of equipment and cleans tray				
Documentation				
Date and time transfusion started				
Date and time transfusion finished				
Reason for transfusion				
Patient consent				
Type of blood product				
Number of units transfused				
Unit and batch numbers				
Outcome of transfusion				
Adverse reactions (if any)				
General Points				
Talks to the patient throughout the procedure				
Avoids patient contamination (i.e. NTT)				

0 = Not attempted
1 = Performed, with room for improvement
2 = Adequately performed
3 = Performed beyond level expected

 Fact Box

Each unit of packed red blood cells is expected to increase the Hb level by approximately 1 g/L.

STATION 3.9: ECGS

SCENARIO

Mr Edmonds, a 70-year-old man, has come to the emergency department (ED) with central crushing chest pain. He has hypertension and is a smoker. An ECG has been performed. Please interpret it and present your findings.

OBJECTIVES

- To learn how to perform an ECG
- To learn how to interpret an ECG
- To learn management of common ECG findings

GENERAL ADVICE

- Obtain consent.

- Remove any body hair over areas where you wish to attach the ECG leads.
- Ensure the patient is lying on a bed, or sitting comfortably, and still.
- Adequately expose the patient. This may involve bra removal in female patients.
- Inform female patients that the chest electrode stickers will be placed underneath their breast.
- Ask the patient if they have any allergies. Patients may be allergic to the electrode sticker adhesive.

PERFORMING AN ECG

There is a universal standard when performing a 12-lead ECG. Six chest leads and four limb leads are attached to the patient. The chest leads are labelled V1—V6 and are positioned as follows (Fig. 3.53):

- V1 — Fourth intercostal space, right sternal edge
- V2 — Fourth intercostal space, left sternal edge
- V3 — Site midway between V2 and V4
- V4 — Fifth intercostal space, mid-clavicular line
- V5 — Fifth intercostal space, anterior axillary line
- V6 — Fifth intercostal space, mid-axillary line

The limb leads are positioned as follows (Fig. 3.54):

- aVR — Right wrist or shoulder (red lead)
- aVL — Left wrist or shoulder (yellow lead)
- aVF — Left ankle (green lead)
- N — Right ankle (black lead)

These leads are attached and generate a 12-lead ECG recording.

RECORDING THE ECG

1. Check the machine's calibration with the 1-mV signal (normally 1 cm = 1 mV).
2. Set the recording speed to 25 mm/s.
3. Wash your hands.
4. Place 10 electrode stickers on the patient's skin in the correct positions, as outlined above.
5. Ensure the electrode stickers are placed with the small tab downwards. This ensures the lead clips will lie flat against the patient's skin.
6. Attach the electrodes to the stickers.
7. Check that all electrode stickers and electrodes are correctly attached to the patient.
8. Ask the patient to remain still and quiet.
9. Press the 'record' button.

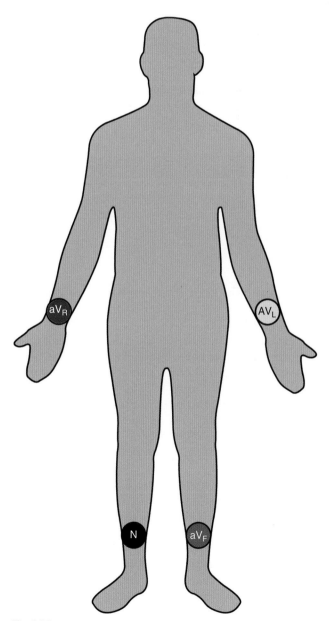

Fig. 3.54 Anatomical position of the ECG limb leads.

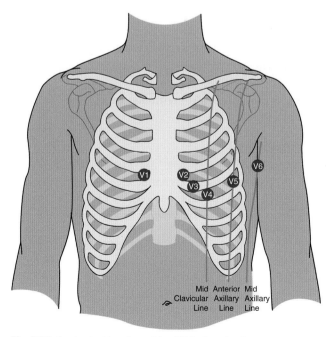

Fig. 3.53 Anatomical location of the ECG chest leads.

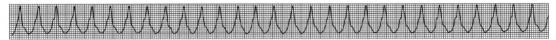

Fig. 3.55 VT (regular rhythm, with broad complexes).

10. Check the printed ECG to ensure that there is a good trace.
11. Repeat the ECG if there is a poor trace.

FINISHING

1. Label the ECG with the patient's details.
2. Remove the electrodes and the electrode stickers from the patient.
3. Ask the patient to get dressed, and offer assistance if required.
4. Document the ECG recording in the notes and interpret it.

INTERPRETING AN ECG

IMPORTANT INFORMATION TO NOTE

- Time and date of ECG
- Patient details (name, date of birth)
- Calibration
- Paper speed – usually 25 mm/s (one small square = 40 ms)
- Heart rate
- Heart rhythm
- Cardiac axis
- Morphology

HEART RATE

First assess if the heart rhythm is regular or irregular.
- If regular, count the number of large boxes between adjacent R waves.
  - Divide this number by 300. For example, if there are three large boxes between R waves, 300/3 = a heart rate of 100 beats/min.
- If irregular, the heart rate may still be roughly estimated. The rhythm strip normally corresponds to 10 s of electrical activity. The number of R waves present in the rhythm strip can therefore be multiplied by 6 to give the number of heart beats each minute.
  - For example, if there were 2 RR intervals on the 10-s rhythm strip, the heart rate is 22 × 6 = 132 beats/min (alternatively, dividing the number of large squares between 3 RR intervals into 900 is another way to calculate irregular rates).
  Normal heart rate is defined as 60–100 beats/min. A heart rate >100 beats/min is defined as tachycardia. A heart rate <60 beats/min is defined as bradycardia.

Note that not all tachycardias and bradycardias are pathological, and they often reflect the physiological state; for example, sleeping, exercising and stress.

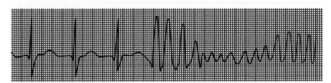

Fig. 3.56 TdP (evolves on the right of this ECG strip — note that the height of the complexes gradually decreases and then increases).

TACHYCARDIA

BROAD-COMPLEX TACHYCARDIA

- VT (Fig. 3.55)
- Torsades de Pointes (TdP) (Fig. 3.56)

MANAGEMENT

Such rhythms of broad-complex tachyarrhythmias are potentially life-threatening and should be managed immediately:
- Resuscitate using an ABC approach (see station 3.1).
- Give oxygen.
- Put out crash call.
- Obtain IV access.
- Identify reversible causes such as electrolyte imbalances.
- The decision to administer direct-current (DC) shock or medication will depend on the haemodynamic status of the patient as well as the type of rhythm identified.

Note: Supraventricular tachycardia (SVT) with aberrant conduction can look like VT. If in doubt, treat as VT.

NARROW-COMPLEX TACHYCARDIA

- SVT (Fig. 3.57)
- Atrial flutter (Fig. 3.58)
- Atrial fibrillation (AF) with fast ventricular response (Fig. 3.59)

MANAGEMENT

- Resuscitate using an ABC approach (see station 3.1).
- If the patient is haemodynamically unstable, put out a crash call as the patient may require DC cardioversion.
- Inform a senior if the patient is stable and does not require a crash team.
- If the rhythm is regular, try vagal manoeuvre:
  - Ask the patient to perform a vagal manoeuvre by blowing into a syringe.
  - Perform carotid sinus massage.
- Consider IV adenosine (6 mg IV using cardiac monitoring with full arrest facilities available in case required).
- If the rhythm is irregularly irregular (AF), a β-blocker or digoxin can be given.

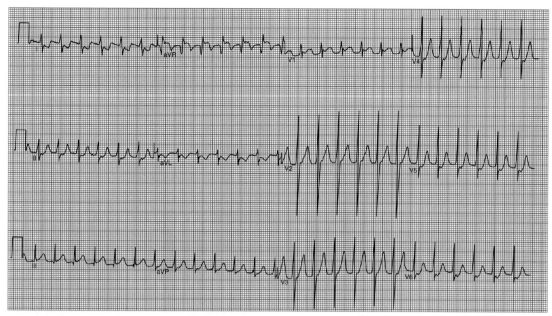

Fig. 3.57 SVT (no P waves seen, narrow complex). (Courtesy of Dr Richard Mansfield)

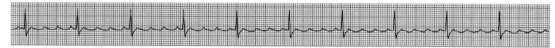

Fig. 3.58 Atrial flutter (saw tooth flutter waves visible, narrow complex, regular).

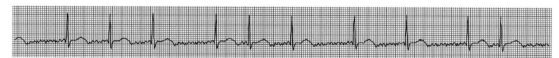

Fig. 3.59 AF (no P waves, narrow complex, irregularly irregular).

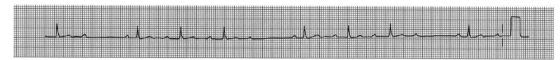

Fig. 3.60 Mobitz type I (the PR interval gradually prolongs until there is a dropped QRS complex).

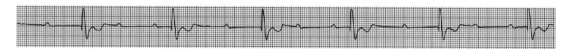

Fig. 3.61 Third-degree heart block (complete disassociation between P waves and QRS complexes). (Courtesy of Dr Richard Mansfield)

BRADYCARDIA

- First-degree heart block — The PR interval is prolonged but there are no dropped beats.
- Second-degree heart block Mobitz type I — The PR interval gradually prolongs until there is a P wave that is not followed by a QRS complex (Fig. 3.60).
- Second-degree heart block Mobitz type II — The PR interval is the same but a QRS is dropped in a regular manner.
- Complete (third-degree) heart block — The P waves and QRS complexes are completely disassociated (Fig. 3.61).

MANAGEMENT

- Carry out resuscitation using an ABC approach (see station 3.1).
- If the patient is haemodynamically stable, then there may be no need to do anything in the acute setting. Identify any medications that may be causing bradycardia, such as β-blockers, and arrange for the patient to be on a cardiac monitor if one is available.
- If the patient is unstable, inform a senior or put out a crash call.
- 500 micrograms (mcg) of atropine should be considered.

- The patient may need transcutaneous or internal pacing as a temporary measure.

Axis	Lead I	Lead aVF
Normal	+	+
Left-axis deviation	+	−
Right-axis deviation	−	+
Extreme right-axis deviation	−	−

Note: This table is a simplification. The most accurate method of determining the axis is to work out the exact angle of the axis. Remember also that a negative aVF, with a positive lead I, can be normal if it is in the zero? to −30 degree range. However, most doctors use this simplification in everyday practice.

CARDIAC AXIS

- The cardiac axis is the overall direction of the wave of ventricular depolarisation (measured in the vertical plane).
- This is measured from a zero reference point (from the same viewpoint as lead I).
- An axis above this line is denoted by a negative number (of degrees), and an axis lying below this line is given a positive number (of degrees).

There are several ways to calculate the axis. Here is the simplest:

A lead is 'positive' if there is a greater positive deflection in the QRS complex than the negative deflection (i.e. the R wave is taller than the S wave). A 'negative' lead has a greater negative deflection.

WAVE MORPHOLOGY

P WAVES

- If all the P waves in the rhythm strip are of similar morphology, it is likely that they are arising from the same focus.
- If tall, consider right atrium enlargement ('P pulmonale').
- If bifid, consider left atrium enlargement ('P mitrale').
- If flattened, consider hyperkalaemia.

QRS COMPLEX

If widened (>120 ms), there is a bundle branch block present. Using the mnemonic 'WILLIAM MARROW' can be helpful:

- WiLLiaM (L for left bundle branch block (LBBB) — WM corresponds to V1 looking like 'W' and V6 looking like 'M'. There are deep S waves in leads V1–3, and tall R waves in V5–6) (Fig. 3.62).
- MaRRoW (R for right bundle branch block (RBBB) — MW corresponds to V1 looking like 'M' and V6 looking like 'W'. There is a second R wave in V1–3, and a wide slurred S wave in lead V5–6 (Fig. 3.63).
- New-onset LBBB in the setting of suspected acute coronary syndrome (ACS) should be managed the same as ST elevated myocardial infarction (STEMI).

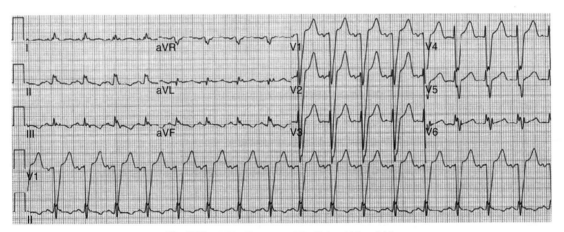

Fig. 3.62 LBBB. (Courtesy of Dr Richard Mansfield)

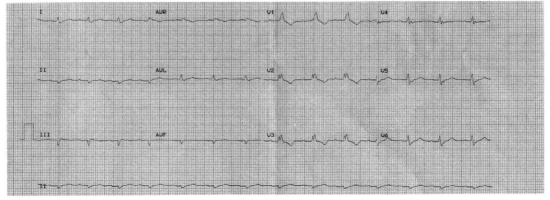

Fig. 3.63 RBBB.

Causes of LBBB	Causes of RBBB
MI	Normal variant
Hypertension	MI
Conduction system fibrosis	Pulmonary embolism
Cardiomyopathy	Cor pulmonale
	Congenital heart disease
	Cardiomyopathy

ST SEGMENTS

The important changes to look for are either elevation or depression. The two important differentials for ST elevation are pericarditis and MI.
Note: In the presence of LBBB, the ST segment cannot be accurately interpreted.

	STEMI	Pericarditis
Site	ST elevation localised to ischaemic territory	Widespread 'saddle-shaped' ST elevation
ST depression	Reciprocal ST depression; for example, ST depression in the anterior territory with an inferior infarct	No reciprocal change
PR segment	Normal	PR depression

Other causes of ST elevation include left ventricular aneurysm. ST elevation may also be confused with early repolarisation. Causes of ST depression include:
- Myocardial ischaemia
- Digoxin ('reverse tick' appearance of ST segment)
- Left/right ventricular hypertrophy
- Bundle branch block
- Hypokalaemia

Q-WAVE CHANGES

A pathological Q wave is one which is greater than one-third of the height of the R wave on the same QRS complex and has a duration of greater than 40 ms. This is suggestive of an old infarct.

In the context of an evolving infarct, if Q waves develop on serial ECGs, this is suggestive of a complete infarct.

T-WAVE CHANGES

The two most important causes of T-wave change are myocardial ischaemia and hyperkalaemia.

Ischaemic T-wave changes
- T-wave inversion (can be normal in V1, III and aVR, especially if present in old ECGs)
- Flattened T waves
- Biphasic T waves
- Peaked T waves

If T-wave inversion occurs across several leads in the same myocardial territory, myocardial ischaemia becomes more likely.

Hyperkalaemia is associated with tall tented T waves.

ISCHAEMIC CHANGES ON ECGS

STEMI
- STEMI corresponds to total coronary artery occlusion.
- ST elevation will be in the lead that corresponds to a particular territory of a coronary artery.
- An important differential for ST elevation is pericarditis. ST elevation in pericarditis is often in all the leads and is saddle shaped.
- Dominant R waves in leads V1–3, with significant ST depression, are suggestive of a posterior STEMI, which is easily missed if not actively looked for.

Management of STEMI
- Resuscitate using an ABC approach (see station 3.1)
- Oxygen to maintain SaO_2 95%–98%
- Sublingual GTN (1–2 puffs) and aspirin (300 mg)
- IV morphine (1–10 mg titrated to pain)
- If available, contact the cardiology emergency team with a view to arranging primary coronary intervention. Consider additional therapies depending on context e.g. prasugrel, clopidogrel, heparin.
- Once stable, the priority is to restore coronary perfusion as soon as possible
- Bloods, including a troponin and clotting

NON-STEMI (NSTEMI)
- T-wave inversion and/or ST depression
- Indicates subtotal occlusion of coronary artery
- NSTEMI can only be diagnosed with the presence of a raised troponin

Management of NSTEMI
- Resuscitate using an ABC approach (see station 3.1)
- Oxygen to maintain SaO_2 95%–98%
- Sublingual glyceryl trinitrate (GTN) (1–2 puffs)
- Aspirin (300 mg)
- Consider ticagrelor or clopidogrel
- Low-molecular-weight heparin or factor Xa inhibitor, e.g. fondaparinux (2.5 mg)
- IV morphine (1–10 mg titrated to pain)
- Blood tests, including troponin and clotting
- Inform a senior
- Serial ECGs

Note: The management of MI may vary between Trusts. Ensure you are familiar with the protocols of the Trust you are working in.

ANATOMICAL RELATIONS OF ECG LEADS

- II, III, aVF: inferior surface (right coronary artery or left circumflex)
- V1, V2, V3, V4: anterior surface (left anterior descending coronary artery)
- I, aVL, V5, V6: lateral surface (left coronary artery, circumflex)
- V5, V6: high lateral leads (left coronary artery, circumflex)

RHYTHM

1. Are normal P waves present?
2. Is each P wave followed by a QRS complex?
   - If yes to both of the above questions, the rhythm is sinus.
3. What is the PR interval (i.e. looking for heart block)?
   - If there are P waves, is the PR interval the same for each QRS complex?
   - Is the PR interval the normal length (3–5 small squares (120–200 ms))?
4. What is the QRS duration?
   - If QRS duration >120 ms ('broach complex'), the focus of an arrhythmia will usually be coming from within the ventricles, for example, VT. If there is a P wave preceding each QRS, it would indicate aberrant conduction due to LBBB, RBBB or ventricular pre-excitation due to Wolff–Parkinson–White syndrome, but the PR interval is short in Wolff–Parkinson–White syndrome.

- A QRS duration <120 ms ('narrow-complex') implies ventricular depolarisation via the His/Purkinje system, which can only occur with a supraventricular focus.

REPORTING AN ECG

- Remember the report has two parts – describing the ECG and interpretng it.
- Follow the same order for each ECG you report:
  - Patient details, date and time of ECG
  - Rate
  - Rhythm
  - Axis
  - P waves and PR interval
  - QRS complexes:
    - Duration
    - Presence of Q waves
    - Height of R and S waves
  - ST segments
  - T waves

Present Your Findings

Mr Edmonds, a 70-year-old man, presented to the ED with central crushing chest pain. An ECG was performed which showed that he was tachycardic at 100 beats/min and in sinus rhythm, normal cardiac axis. ST elevations were seen across leads V5 and V6. P waves, PR interval, QRS complexes and T waves were unremarkable. He is currently being treated as a STEMI and has had sublingual GTN, 300 mg aspirin and 300 mg clopidogrel. The cardiology team has been contacted, and we are currently awaiting his first troponin level to return from the laboratory as well.

Mark Scheme for Examiner

	0	1	2	3
General				
Checks patient details and date/time of the ECG				
Notes paper speed				
Interpretation and Presenting				
Comments on rate				
Comments on rhythm				
Comments on axis				
Comments on P-wave morphology				
Comments on PR interval				
Comments on QRS morphology				
Comments on ST segment				
Comments on T waves				
Comments on Q waves				
Presents findings				
Concludes and interprets findings with consideration of patient's symptoms				

0 = Not attempted
1 = Performed, with room for improvement
2 = Adequately performed
3 = Performed beyond level expected

❓ QUESTIONS AND ANSWERS FOR CANDIDATE

What are the two types of second-degree heart block, and which is more worrying?

- Mobitz type 1 or Wenckebach heart block is when there is a lengthening of each PR interval, until a QRS is 'dropped' for a non-conducted P wave.
- Mobitz type 2 is when the PR interval is constant, but occasionally there is no QRS wave, i.e. the P wave is not conducted. Mobitz type 2 is the more worrying type of second-degree heart block as it can turn into third-degree heart block, when there is no association between P and QRS waves.

What is the difference between VF and VT on an ECG?

How would AF be diagnosed from ECG findings?

- Irregularly irregular rhythm
- Absence of P waves (chaotic baseline due to atria fibrillating)
- QRS <120 s
- Heart rate can be normal, especially if the patient is on treatment

What is an ectopic beat?

- Ectopic beats are changes in a heart beat, that is otherwise normal, that often lead to a skipped or missed heart beat.

What are the most common types of ectopic beats?

- Premature atrial contraction (PAC)
- Premature ventricular contraction (PVC)

Ventricular Tachycardia (VT)	Ventricular Fibrillation (VF)
Regular rhythm	Irregular rhythm
QRS complex >120 s	QRS complex >120 s
P waves may be present but there is no relationship with QRS complexes. There is no association between atrial and ventricular activity	P waves absent

EXAMPLE ECGS (TABLE 3.2)

〜 Table 3.2   Interpretations of example ECGs

EXAMPLE NUMBER	BACKGROUND	RATE, RHYTHM, AXIS	MORPHOLOGY	SUMMARY
1	This is an ECG of Mr Fredrickson, a 65-year-old male, who is currently asymptomatic, and haemodynamically stable	The heart rate is 94 bpm, the rhythm is regular. The axis is within normal limits	P waves are present, the PR interval is normal, QRS complexes are narrow, and there are no ST or T wave changes	In summary, this ECG is consistent with sinus rhythm
2	This is an ECG of Mr Fredrickson, a 65-year-old male, who is currently asymptomatic and haemodynamically stable	The heart rate is 84 (14 × 6) beats/min, the rhythm is irregularly irregular. The axis is within normal limits	No P waves are present. QRS complexes are narrow, and there are no ST- or T-wave changes	In summary, this ECG is consistent with AF
3	This is an ECG of Mr Fredrickson, a 65-year-old male, who is currently asymptomatic and haemodynamically stable	The heart rate is 138 beats/min, the rhythm is regular. This axis is within normal limits	P waves have a saw-toothed appearance, and there are two per QRS complex, which are	In summary, this ECG is consistent with atrial flutter

Continued

Table **3.2** Interpretations of example ECGs—cont'd

EXAMPLE NUMBER	BACKGROUND	RATE, RHYTHM, AXIS	MORPHOLOGY	SUMMARY
			narrow. There are no ST- or T-wave changes	
4	This is an ECG of Mr Fredrickson, a 65-year-old male, who presented with an episode of chest pain, and collapse. He is haemodynamically stable	The heart rate is 42 beats/min, the rhythm is regular. This axis is within normal limits	P waves are present, but there is no relationship with QRS complexes, which are narrow. There is 1 mm ST elevation in leads II, III and aVF, and 1 mm of ST depression in aVL. There is T-wave inversion in I, AVL and aVR. There are biphasic T waves in V1—4	In summary, this ECG is consistent with complete heart block. The ST-and T-wave changes may represent a ventricular escape rhythm morphology OR an inferior MI causing sinoatrial node ischaemia, and subsequent heart block
5	This is an ECG of Mr Fredrickson, a 65-year-old male, who is currently suffering from chest pain, but is haemodynamically stable	The heart rate is 82 beats/min, the rhythm is regular. This axis is within normal limits	P waves are present, PR interval is normal and QRS complexes are narrow. There is massive ST elevation, up to 16 mm, in leads I, aVL, V2—6 and T-wave inversion in lead aVL. There is ST depression in leads II, III and aVF. Four ectopics are also present	In summary, this ECG is consistent with an anterolateral STEMI, with reciprocal inferior ST depression
6	This is an ECG of Mr. Fredrickson, a 65-year-old male, who is currently suffering from palpitations, and has a peripheral pulse of 253 beats/min, and a BP of 92/60 mmHg	The heart rate is 260 beats/min, the rhythm is regular. This axis is within normal limits	P waves are not clearly visible (although if you look carefully, they can be seen buried in the T wave), and QRS complexes are narrow. There is ST depression (up to 5 mm) in leads I, II, aVF and V4—6	In summary, this ECG is consistent with SVT, with probable rate-related inferolateral ischaemia
7	This is an ECG of Mr. Fredrickson, a 65-year-old male, who has had a cardiac arrest	The heart rate is 300 beats/min, the rhythm is regular. This axis is within normal limits	P waves are not clearly visible, and QRS complexes are wide. ST segment and T-wave changes cannot be seen	In summary, this ECG is consistent with a broad-complex tachycardia (either VT or SVT with bundle branch block)

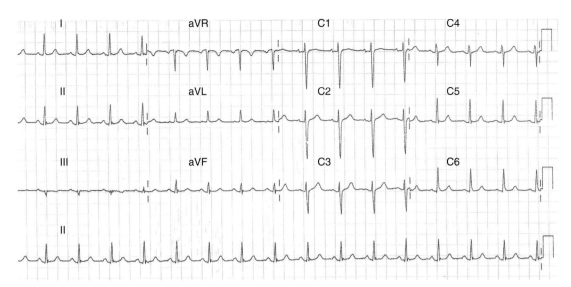

Example 1 This is an ECG of Mr Fredrickson, a 65-year-old male, who is currently asymptomatic, and haemodynamically stable.

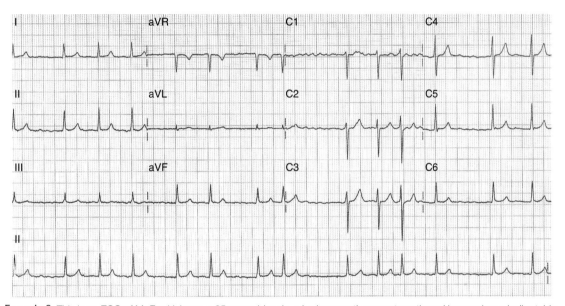

Example 2 This is an ECG of Mr Fredrickson, a 65-year-old male, who is currently asymptomatic and haemodynamically stable.

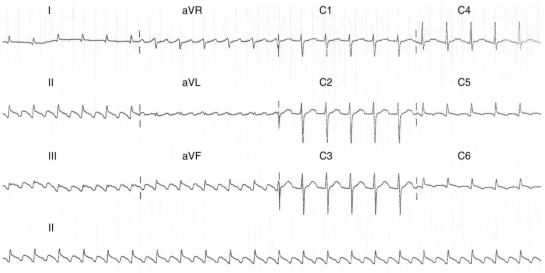

Example 3 This is an ECG of Mr Fredrickson, a 65-year-old male, who is currently asymptomatic and haemodynamically stable.

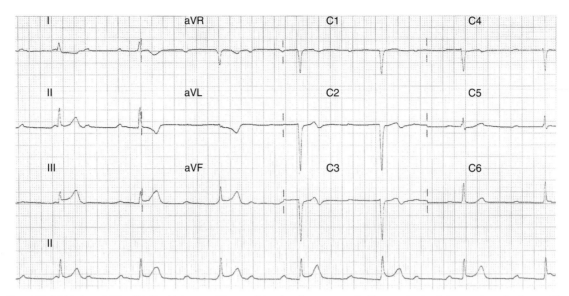

Example 4 This is an ECG of Mr Fredrickson, a 65-year-old male, who presented with an episode of chest pain and collapse. He is haemodynamically stable.

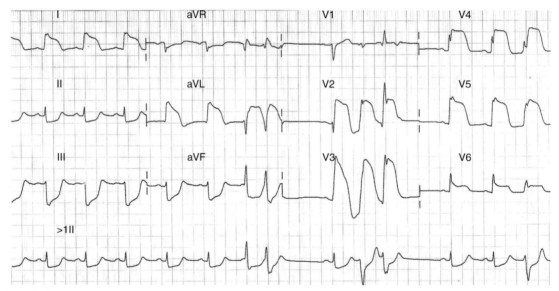

Example 5 This is an ECG of Mr Fredrickson, a 65-year-old male, who is currently suffering from chest pain, but is haemodynamically stable.

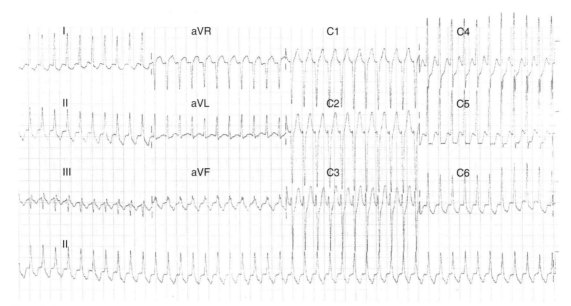

Example 6 This is an ECG of Mr. Fredrickson, a 65-year-old male, who is currently suffering from palpitations, and has a peripheral pulse of 253 beats/min, and a BP of 92/60 mmHg. (Courtesy of Pamela Gulland/Hannah Collinson)

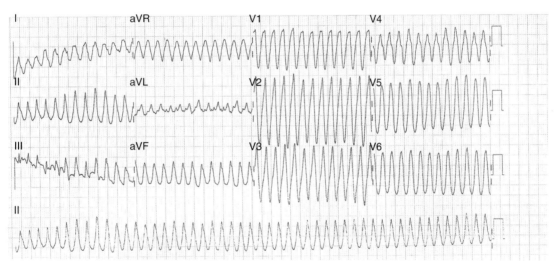

Example 7 This is an ECG of Mr. Fredrickson, a 65-year-old male, who has had a cardiac arrest.

Tip Box

Always try and compare a new ECG against an old one so that acute changes are more obvious and chronic abnormalities are not taken as new changes. It can sometimes be difficult to differentiate between true ST segment elevation and 'high take off' of the ST segment into the T wave. It is always important to correlate the ECG with the patient's symptoms and, if in doubt, seek a second opinion from a senior colleague.

Fact Box

The J (Osborn) wave is positive deflection at the J point and is characteristically seen in hypothermia. However, they are not pathognomonic.

STATION 3.10: FUNDOSCOPY

SCENARIO

Mr Dean is a 62-year-old man with diabetes. He has attended for his annual eye review. Please examine his fundi.

OBJECTIVES

- To learn how to perform fundoscopy
- To learn how to interpret common findings on fundoscopy

GENERAL ADVICE

- Introduce yourself, explain what fundoscopy involves and obtain consent.
- Explanation to the patient should include you informing them that you will have to come closer to their head during the examination.
- Dilate the pupils if necessary, using dilating drops. Tropicamide is frequently used as it is short-acting (4−6 h).
- Check the ophthalmoscope settings.

EQUIPMENT CHECKLIST

- Ophthalmoscope

FUNDOSCOPY

POSITIONING

- Have the patient sitting in a dark room.
- Dilate the pupils.
- To examine the right eye, use your right hand and right eye, and vice versa (Fig. 3.64).
- Keep your index finger on the dial at the side of the ophthalmoscope so you can adjust the focus if needed whilst examining. It may help to start on a low 'plus' setting, and ratchet anticlockwise towards minus until the image is clear (minus, anti-clockwise, corrects for myopia).
- 'O' is the equivalent of no refractive error, negative red numbers correct for myopic (short-sighted), and positive green numbers correct for hypermetropic (long-sighted).

EXAMINATION SEQUENCE

Red reflex

1. Before moving in to see the fundus, look for the red reflex from approximately 30 cm, at approximately a 45-degree angle to the nose.
2. Incomplete/absent red reflex: Think cataracts, corneal opacities or tumours.

Optic disc

1. Find a large vessel and trace it back to find the optic disc (Fig. 3.65).
2. Assess the:
   - Optic disc colour (i.e. pale in optic atrophy)
   - Disc margin (i.e. blurred in papilloedema)
   - Cup (i.e. increased cup:disc ratio in glaucoma)

Macula

1. Look for abnormalities in this area, i.e. haemorrhages or exudates in diabetic maculopathy.

Vessels

1. Trace the four major vessel arcs out to the periphery.
2. Veins appear darker than arteries.
3. Look for:
   - Arteriovenous (AV) nipping (at vessel crossing points); for example, in hypertension
   - Haemorrhages or vessel tortuosity; for example, in diabetes or hypertension
   - Microaneurysms; for example, in diabetes
   - Silver wiring; for example, in hypertension

Periphery

1. Examine each quadrant, ensuring that the retina looks pink and healthy.

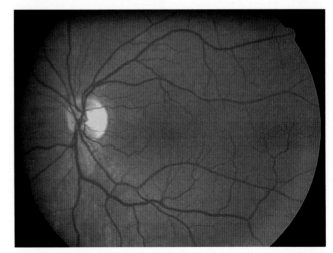

Fig. 3.65 A healthy eye. Note the clear margins of the optic disc. (Courtesy of NHS Fife)

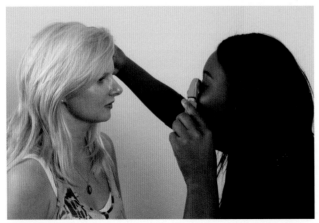

Fig. 3.64 Ensure correct positioning when examining the patient.

2. Due to the magnification of the ophthalmoscope, it is difficult to visualise the periphery.

DIABETIC RETINOPATHY

- The main risk factor for diabetic retinopathy is the length of time the person has had diabetes.
- All patients with diabetes should be screened for retinopathy at least annually.
- Incidence is lower with excellent glycaemic control.

NON-PROLIFERATIVE DIABETIC RETINOPATHY (NPDR) (FIG. 3.66)

- Microaneurysms (smaller and more distinct than dot haemorrhage, but it is difficult to differentiate between the two)
- Dot and blot haemorrhages
- Hard exudates
- Cotton-wool spots (due to local ischaemia)
- Normal visual acuity
- No treatment indicated, only regular follow-up

SEVERE NON-PROLIFERATIVE DIABETIC RETINOPATHY

- Venous beading/dilatation/tortuosity
- Larger and more widespread blot haemorrhages
- Intraretinal microvascular abnormality
- Closer follow-up

PROLIFERATIVE DIABETIC RETINOPATHY

- Neovascularisation (due to ischaemia): new vessels on the disc or elsewhere
- Risk of vitreous haemorrhage (new vessels are friable and prone to bleeding, particularly those close to the disc)
- Risk of tractional retinal detachment

- Severe loss of vision may occur secondary to these; neovascularisation is an indication for urgent referral for photocoagulation

DIABETIC MACULOPATHY

- Vessel leakage and/or ischaemia at the macula
- Most common cause of visual loss in diabetes

LASER TREATMENT SCARS

- Panretinal photocoagulation (PRP) is used for proliferative diabetic retinopathy
- Focal/grid laser photocoagulation is used for diabetic maculopathy

HYPERTENSIVE RETINOPATHY (FIG. 3.67)

- Arteriolar narrowing
- AV nipping at crossing points
- Copper or silver wiring (increased central light reflex from arterioles)
- Cotton-wool spots
- Hard exudates, which may surround the macula forming a partial or complete 'star'
- Blot or flame haemorrhages
- Usually asymptomatic if chronic

ACCELERATED HYPERTENSION

- Disc swelling, indicating an optic neuropathy, as well as retinopathy changes above
- May have reduced visual acuity
- Usually severe hypertension (e.g. systolic BP >220 mmHg) and evidence of other end-organ damage

PAPILLOEDEMA (FIG. 3.68)

- Bilateral disc swelling secondary to raised intra-cranial pressure
- Blurred disc margin ± disc pallor

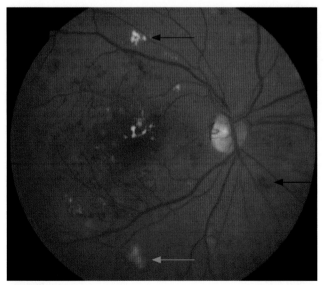

Fig. 3.66 Features of NRDR: dot and blot haemorrhages (black arrow), hard exudates (blue arrow) and cotton-wool spots (green arrow). (Courtesy of NHS Lothian)

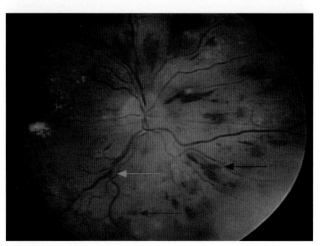

Fig. 3.67 Features of hypertensive retinopathy: blot (blue arrow) and flame-shaped haemorrhages (black arrow); AV nipping (green arrow). (Courtesy of Dr Ed Friedlander)

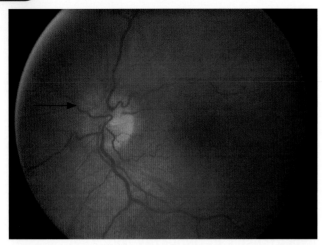

Fig. 3.68 Features of papilloedema: blurred margins (black arrow), which indicate a swollen optic disc. (Courtesy of NHS Fife)

- If long-standing, you may see dilated veins and hard exudates

OPTIC NEURITIS
- Inflammation or demyelination

ANTERIOR ISCHAEMIC OPTIC NEUROPATHY
- Infarction of the optic nerve head, usually secondary to giant cell arteritis (GCA) and hypertension

AGE-RELATED MACULAR DEGENERATION (AMD)
- Commonest cause of blindness in the developed world for the over-50s

DRY (ATROPHIC) AMD (FIG. 3.69)
- Degeneration at and around the macula. More common than wet AMD
- Atrophic (pale) ± hyperpigmented areas

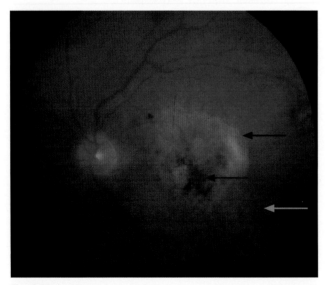

Fig. 3.69 Features of dry AMD: pale area around the macula (black arrow), hyperpigmented areas (blue arrow) and soft drusen (green arrow). (Courtesy of NHS Lothian)

- Drusen (subretinal deposits of waste products)
- No treatment

WET (NEOVASCULAR) AMD
- Choroidal neovascularisation, which may leak, leading to oedema and haemorrhage
- More rapid loss of vision
- Antivascular endothelial growth factor (VEGF) injections into the vitreous or sometimes laser treatment may be given

🔍 Present Your Findings

Mr Dean is a 62-year-old man with a history of diabetes for 30 years. On fundoscopic examination, there is evidence of venous tortuosity and more widespread blot haemorrhages. This is in keeping with severe NPDR. I would like to complete my examination by performing a slit-lamp examination, and discussing with Mr Dean how well controlled his diabetes is and whether further investigations are required. I would also like to check for other macrovascular complications of diabetes; for example, neuropathy and nephropathy.

❓ QUESTIONS AND ANSWERS FOR CANDIDATE

What are the differential diagnoses of a 'red eye'?
- Subconjunctival haemorrhage
- Conjunctivitis
- Glaucoma
- Anterior uveitis
- Scleritis/episcleritis

Name three causes of a relative afferent pupil defect (RAPD).
- Optic neuritis
- Optic atrophy
- Papillitis
- Retinal detachment
- Central retinal artery occlusion (CRAO)
- Widespread retinal disease
- Optic nerve compression

What may you see in a third-nerve palsy?
- The affected eye appears outwards and downwards
- Ptosis of the upper eyelid
- Diplopia
- Fixed and dilated pupil
- Only lateral movement is possible; the patient cannot move the eye in vertical motions

What is the difference between scleritis and episcleritis?
- Scleritis is inflammation involving the sclera, whereas episcleritis is inflammation of the superficial episclera, the layer between the conjunctiva and the sclera. The main differentiating symptom between the two is that episcleritis usually presents with minimal pain, whereas scleritis is a severe, dull, boring pain.

Mark Scheme for Examiner

	0	1	2	3
Introduction and General Preparation				
Introduces self, and washes hands				
Confirms patient's identity with three points of identification				
Explains procedure, identifies concerns and obtains consent				
Warns the patient about the need to be close to their face				
Positioning and Technique				
Darkens room, and asks patient to sit				
Dilates pupils if needed				
Uses orrect technique in adjustment of ophthalmoscope				
Uses correct hand to hold ophthalmoscope when examining				
Examination				
Elicits the red reflex				
Examines the optic disc				
Examines the macula				
Examines the peripheries in all four quadrants				
Reports findings appropriately				
Explains findings to patient				

0 = Not attempted
1 = Performed, with room for improvement
2 = Adequately performed
3 = Performed beyond level expected

How does blepharitis present?

- Blepharitis is inflammation of the eyelids, and it can present with:
  - Red eyes or eyelids
  - Gritty sensation in the eyes
  - Itchy eyes
  - Painful eyelids
  - Sticky eyelids
  - Crusts around the roots of the eyelashes

 Tip Box

Dilating drops can blur the patient's vision and therefore you must make them aware of this, and make sure they do not drive until their vision has returned to normal.

 Fact Box

Signs of thyroid eye disease include:
- Lid retraction (Dalrymple's sign)
- Lid lag on downgaze (von Graefe's sign)
- Exophthalmos (proptosis) due to oedema of extraocular muscles
- Restricted extraocular movements
- Chemosis (conjunctival oedema)

STATION 3.11: OTOSCOPY

SCENARIO

Mr Downing is an 82-year-old man complaining of difficulty hearing the television over the last few months. Please perform an otoscopic examination to evaluate the cause of his hearing loss.

OBJECTIVES

- To learn how to perform otoscopy
- To learn how to interpret common findings on otoscopy

GENERAL ADVICE

- Introduce yourself, explain what otoscopy involves and obtain consent.
- Explanation to the patient should include you informing them that you will have to place a speculum within the ear canal during the examination.
- Check the otoscope lighting.

EQUIPMENT CHECKLIST

- Clean disposable speculum (one for each ear)
- Otoscope

OTOSCOPY

EXAMINATION SEQUENCE

1. Select a 4-mm speculum and attach it to the otoscope.
2. Turn the otoscope to full brightness.
3. Hold the otoscope and place your little finger on the patient's zygoma to ensure you have full control of the otoscope at all times.
4. Lift the pinna upwards and backwards with your other hand (Fig. 3.70).
5. Place the speculum on the posterior aspect of the tragus, and then carefully insert the speculum into the ear canal whilst looking through the otoscope
   - Examine the external auditory meatus
   - Take note of any evidence of infection or wax build-up within the ear canal
   - Try to identify the different parts of the tympanic membrane, and make note of any abnormalities seen.
6. Repeat the examination with the other ear.

OTOSCOPY IMAGES

Refer to Figs 3.71–3.76

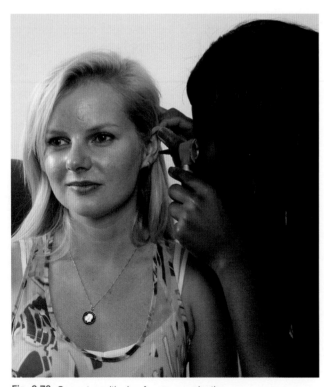

Fig. 3.70 Correct positioning for ear examination.

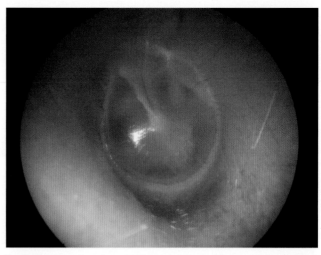

Fig. 3.71 Normal anatomy of the tympanic membrane. (Courtesy of Dr David Pothier (www.earatlas.co.uk))

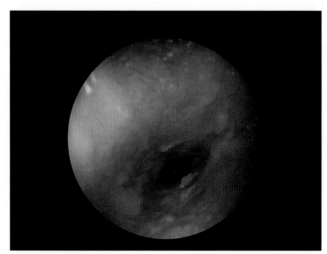

Fig. 3.72 Acute otitis externa. (Courtesy of Dr David Pothier (www.earatlas.co.uk))

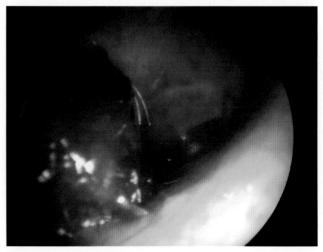

Fig. 3.73 Ear wax within the ear canal. (Courtesy of Dr David Pothier (www.earatlas.co.uk))

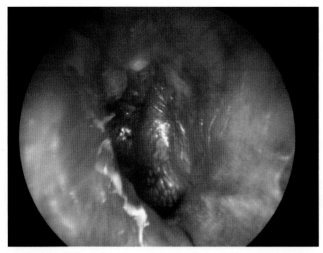

Fig. 3.74 Acute otitis media. (Courtesy of Dr David Pothier (www.earatlas.co.uk))

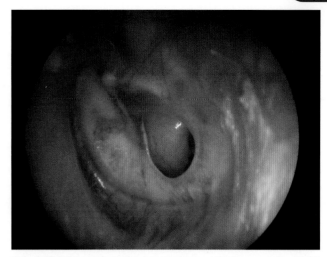

Fig. 3.76 Perforated tympanic membrane. (Courtesy of Dr David Pothier (www.earatlas.co.uk))

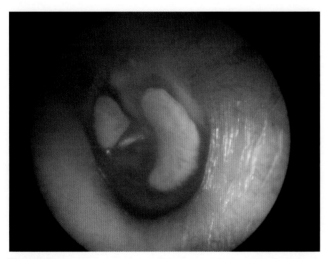

Fig. 3.75 Tympanosclerosis. (Courtesy of Dr David Pothier (www.earatlas.co.uk))

Present Your Findings

Mr Downing is an 82-year-old man presenting with progressive hearing loss over the past 3 months. On otoscopic examination, there is hard brownish-yellow cerumen that obscures the tympanic membrane and appears to be impacted on both sides. This is most likely to be the cause of Mr Downing's hearing loss, but I would like to complete my examination by performing Rinne's and Weber's test and reassess Mr Downing's hearing once the ear wax has been removed.

? QUESTIONS AND ANSWERS FOR CANDIDATE

What factors predispose someone to the development of acute otitis externa?
- Absence of ear wax
- High humidity
- Water in the ear canal
- Trauma due to cotton swabs or hearing aids

What are the indications for the removal of ear wax?
- Total occlusion of the ear canal causing hearing loss, earache or tinnitus
- When direct visualisation of the tympanic membrane is required for diagnostic purposes
- In order to take an impression of the ear canal for a hearing aid mould, or if wax is causing the aid to whistle

What are the complications of otitis media?
- Hearing loss
- Tympanic membrane perforation
- Chronic otitis media with or without cholesteatoma
- Cholesteatoma
- Mastoiditis
- Tympanosclerosis
- Labyrinthitis

What is cholesteatoma, and what is the most important risk factor?
- Cholesteatomas are abnormal growths of skin cells within the ear, behind the ear drum.

Mark Scheme for Examiner

	0	1	2	3
Introduction and General Preparation				
Introduces self, and washes hands				
Confirms patient's identity with three points of identification				
Explains procedure, identifies concerns and obtains consent				
Warns the patient about the need to place a speculum within the ear canal				
Positioning and Technique				
Stabilises hand by resting the little finger on the patient's zygoma				
Carefully places the speculum onto the tragus and then into the ear canal				
Examination				
Examines the ear canal and describes any abnormalities present				
Examines the tympanic membrane and describes any abnormalities present				
Uses a clean speculum for examination of the other ear				
Reports findings appropriately				
Explains findings to patient				

0 = Not attempted
1 = Performed, with room for improvement
2 = Adequately performed
3 = Performed beyond level expected

- They are most commonly caused by repetitive episodes of otitis media.

What is tympanosclerosis, and how is it treated?
- Tympansclerosis is scarring of the ear drum, usually after injury or surgery.
- Depending on the signs and symptoms, it can be treated through surgical intervention.

 Tip Box

Look into as many ears as possible. When you are used to what 'normal' looks like, it will be easier for you to identify the 'abnormal' ears.

 Fact Box

There are a few congenital deformities of the ears that you should be aware of:
- Anotia: Complete absence of the pinna
- Microtia: Underdevelopment of the pinna
- Low-set ear: Ears are positioned at a lower level on the head compared to normal

STATION 3.12: CENTRAL VENOUS LINES

SCENARIO

Mr Arnold is a 30-year-old man with known chronic liver disease who has presented acutely with haematemesis. He is a known IV drug user. As the junior doctor on call, you are asked to see him and after determining that he is physiologically stable, you attempt to cannulate him in order to obtain blood samples and to administer IV fluids. Whilst you struggle to find a peripheral vein suitable for cannulation, Mr Arnold vomits a large volume of fresh blood and becomes haemodynamically unstable. You call for help, and after further attempts at peripheral venous access fail, your registrar prepares to insert a central line. Discuss with the examiner the indications for this procedure, key aspects of insertion and how this procedure might guide fluid resuscitation.

OBJECTIVES

- Be able to recall the indications for central venous cannulation
- Know the general principles of insertion technique
- Be familiar with the concept of central venous pressure (CVP) monitoring

GENERAL ADVICE

- Inserting a central venous catheter (or central line) is a complex procedure and as such you would not be expected to perform it as a junior doctor without instruction from an experienced senior colleague.
- Central venous cannulation involves the insertion of a catheter into the internal jugular vein or subclavian vein (Fig. 3.77).
- There are several indications for central venous cannulation:
  - Poor peripheral venous access
  - CVP monitoring
  - Total parenteral nutrition infusion
  - Inotropic or vasoactive drug infusion
  - Chemotherapy
  - Haemodialysis
- There are numerous, different types of central venous catheter:

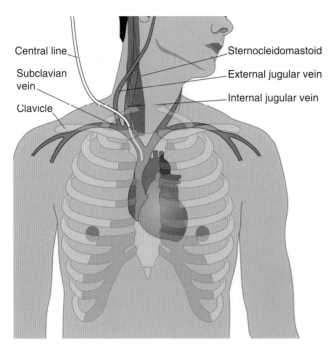

Fig. 3.77 Anatomical diagram of the major vessels involved in central line insertion.

- Tunnelled and non-tunnelled (tunnelled for more long-term use)
- Implantable ports
- Peripherally inserted central catheters (PICCs)
- Dialysis catheters (vascath)
- These, in turn, may be single-lumen or multi-lumen catheters, depending on the intended use of the central line (e.g. a multi-lumen catheter would allow several drugs to be infused and CVP to be monitored simultaneously).

EQUIPMENT CHECKLIST

(Remember to check expiry dates on all equipment (Fig. 3.78).)
- Procedure trolley with sterile drape and swabs
- Sharps bin
- Sterile gown

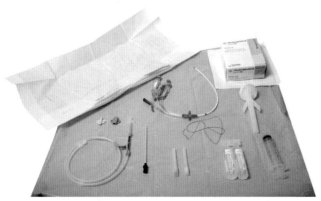

Fig. 3.78 Ensure you have all the equipment you require before heading to the bedside.

- Sterile gloves
- Skin-cleansing solution (e.g. chlorhexidine)
- 10-mL syringe
- 25-gauge and 21-gauge needles
- 10 mL 1% lidocaine
- Seldinger central venous line pack
- Ultrasound machine
- Suture and suturing equipment
- 0.9% saline (for priming and flushing central line)
- Sterile dressing
- Scalpel

Note: Skin-cleansing solutions and method will vary depending on local policy. If taking blood cultures, blood culture bottle ports will need to be fully cleaned and allowed to dry fully before use.

PERFORMING CENTRAL VENOUS CANNULATION (INTERNAL JUGULAR VEIN (IJV))

As mentioned previously, insertion of a central venous catheter is a complex procedure. The following is intended as a brief and simplified explanation to enable you to discuss the broad concepts:

1. The clinician introduces themselves, checks patient identification and obtains informed consent (if possible).
2. The correct equipment is arranged on a clean procedure trolley and checked for faults and expiry dates.
3. The patient is positioned appropriately (supine with a slight head-down tilt of the bed and head turned away from the procedure site).
4. The clinician washes their hands, and puts on the sterile gown and gloves.
5. The central line is primed with saline.
6. The skin is sterilised and draped.
7. The IJV is located using either:
   - Ultrasound guidance (recommended first line)
   - Surface anatomy markings (about the junction of the heads of sternocleidomastoid muscle)
8. Lidocaine is infiltrated into the tissues overlying the cannulation site.
9. The introducer needle is then inserted and the IJV located by aspirating whilst advancing. As soon as flashback is seen, the needle is within the IJV and cannulation is performed using the Seldinger technique (Fig. 3.79).
10. Once the central venous catheter is in situ it can be flushed with saline.
11. The external cuff of the central line can then be secured in place by suturing.
12. A sterile dressing is then applied.

FINISHING

1. Safely dispose of sharps and waste.
2. Document the procedure in the patient's notes.
3. A chest X-ray should be requested in order to:

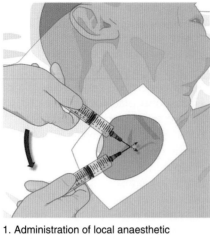

1. Administration of local anaesthetic

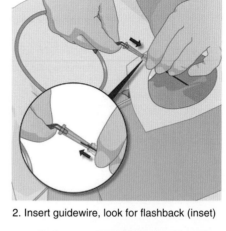

2. Insert guidewire, look for flashback (inset)

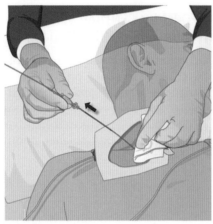

3. Remove cannula

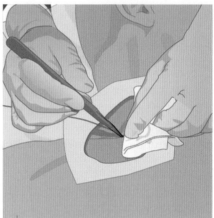

4. Use a scalpel to widen the entry site

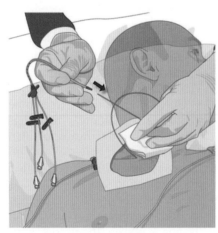

5. Introduce central line catheter

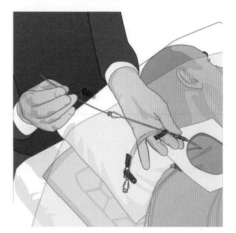

6. Remove guidewire

Fig. 3.79 These steps provide an outline to the Seldinger technique.

- Ensure correct positioning (the tip of the central line will have a radiopaque band. This should appear on a chest X-ray within the superior vena cava at the level of T4/carina)
- Exclude iatrogenic pneumothorax

DOCUMENT THE PROCEDURE

Document under the following headings:
- Central venous line inserted
- Date, time and place

- Indications for the central venous line
- Patient consent
- Whether ultrasound guidance was used
- Local anaesthetic used, volume, expiry date and batch number
- Complications
- Subsequent tests ordered, if any, e.g. chest X-ray

What is a PICC line?

- PICC stands for peripherally inserted central catheter.

Which central veins can be used for catheter insertion?

- Internal jugular
- Subclavian
- Femoral
- Basilic
- Brachial

Which type of line can you not use for dialysis?

- You must *never* use a PICC line for dialysis treatment due to the smaller size and flow rate of these catheters.

Mark Scheme for Examiner

	0	1	2	3
Introduction and General Preparation				
Introduces self, and washes hands				
Confirms patient's identity with three points of identification				
Explains procedure, identifies concerns and obtains consent				
Checks allergies				
Performing Central Venous Cannulation				
Obtains equipment and checks expiry dates				
Positions and prepares patient				
Washes hands, and puts on sterile gown/gloves				
Prepares equipment. Primes central line with saline. Cleans site				
Locates internal jugular vein				
Administers local anaesthesia				
Inserts introducer				
Passes a guidewire				
Removes introducer				
Enlarges puncture site				
Threads catheter				
Removes guidewire				
Flushes catheter and secures using sutures				
Places dressing				
Finishing				
Tells the patient to inform a member of staff if they feel unwell or have any problems with the insertion site				
Disposes of equipment, and cleans tray				
Removes gloves, and washes hands Requests chest X-ray				
Documents procedure in patient notes				
General Points				
Talks continuously to the patient throughout the procedure				
Ensures patient comfort				

0 = Not attempted
1 = Performed, with room for improvement
2 = Adequately performed
3 = Performed beyond level expected

QUESTIONS AND ANSWERS FOR CANDIDATE

Name three indications for the use of central lines.

- Administration of inotropes
- Monitoring CVP
- Long-term drug administration (for example, antibiotics or analgesia)
- Long-term parenteral nutrition
- Chemotherapy

Name three complications of central venous cannulation (specific to the IJV).

- Pneumothorax
- Accidental puncture of the carotid artery
- Haemothorax
- Cardiac arrhythmia
- Catheter blockage
- Infection
- Thrombosis or air embolus
- Injury to nerve roots
- Damage to the stellate ganglion (and subsequent Horner's syndrome)

> **Tip Box**
>
> Before you begin the procedure, confirm what the central venous line is to be used for and how many infusions are required so that you can choose the line with the most appropriate number of lumens.

 Fact Box

CVP monitoring

One use of central venous cannulation is to allow for the measurement of CVP. A specialised catheter tipped with an electrical transducer is passed through the central line and sited in the lower third of the superior vena cava. This allows for continuous real-time measurement of CVP, which is displayed as a characteristic waveform on the cardiac monitor. A normal pressure is 0.8 cm H_2O. As CVP is an accurate measurement of the pressures within the vena cava and right atrium, it can be used as a surrogate marker for cardiac preload. A key use of this is to guide IV fluid therapy — whilst standard arterial BP measurement is useful, CVP measurement better represents the fluid status of the patient. In combination with administering a fluid challenge (rapid administration of ~500 mL of IV crystalloid), the clinician can determine whether the patient's cardiac output can be improved with further fluid administration.

GUIDELINES

Resuscitation Council UK, 2021. Adult advanced life support guidelines. Available at: https://www.resus.org.uk/library/2021-resuscitation-guidelines/adult-advanced-life-support-guidelines (accessed 8 June 2022).

JPAC, 2021. UK blood transfusion and tissue transplantation services. Available at. www.transfusionguidelines.org/ (accessed 8 June 2022).

Medication Administration

Outline

STATION 4.1: INTRAMUSCULAR INJECTIONS

SCENARIO

Mrs Jonas is a 48-year-old woman in the emergency department, who has been suffering with vomiting for the last 6 h. She vomits every time she takes anything orally. You have been asked to administer prescribed intramuscular (IM) cyclizine as she has no intravenous (IV) access.

OBJECTIVE

- To understand how to administer IM injections correctly

GENERAL ADVICE

- When administering any injection, it is important to ensure that the patient has no known drug allergies, that you obtain verbal consent and that you wear gloves.
- When determining the site for the injections, avoid areas showing broken skin, infection, inflammation or swelling.
- If a patient needs daily injections, remember to rotate the injection site to avoid skin irritation, lipo-hypertrophy, lipoatrophy or lipodystrophy.
- Remember to check the expiry date on all equipment.

EQUIPMENT CHECKLIST

(Remember to check expiry dates on all equipment [Fig. 4.1].)
- Tray
- Non-sterile gloves
- Single-use disposable apron
- Skin-cleansing solution
- 21–23-gauge needle
- 21-gauge needle or filter needle for drawing up medication
- Medication for injection
- Syringe (size depending on injection)
- Sharps bin
- Sterile gauze

EXPLAINING INTRAMUSCULAR INJECTION TO THE PATIENT

1. We need to give you some medication into your muscles.

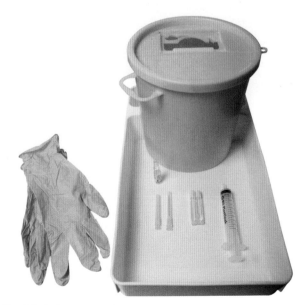

Fig. 4.1 Gather your equipment.

2. A small needle connected to a syringe will be inserted into one of the muscles in your arm.
3. It will be slightly painful.
4. The syringe contains your medication, which will be injected into your muscle so that it can go into your body system.

PREPARATION FOR ALL INJECTIONS

1. Obtain consent.
2. Wash hands and don a pair of non-sterile gloves.

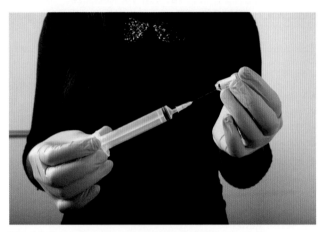

Fig. 4.2 Carefully draw up the medication into a syringe.

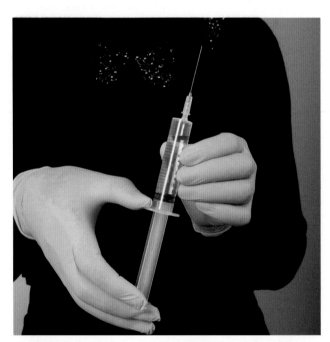

Fig. 4.3 After drawing up medication, check that all the air bubbles have been expelled.

3. Inspect the proposed site for injection and ensure it is suitable.
4. Clean site following local policy. Allow to dry fully.
5. With a colleague, check the drug dose against the drug chart and check the drug expiry date.
6. Draw up the medication using a syringe and a 21-gauge needle if using a plastic ampoule, or a filter needle if using a glass ampoule (Fig. 4.2).
7. Expel any excess air in the syringe (Fig. 4.3).

INTRAMUSCULAR INJECTION

1. Discard the 21-gauge needle in the sharps bin and replace it with a new 21–23-gauge needle.
2. Stabilise the skin around the injection.
3. Hold the syringe like a pencil between your thumb and forefinger.
4. Insert the needle at 90° into the injection site (Fig. 4.4).
5. Draw back in the syringe for 5 s to check that the needle has not penetrated a vein:
   - If there is no flashback, then proceed.
   - If there is flashback, withdraw the needle slightly and recheck for flashback.
6. Slowly inject the medication at a rate in accordance with the instructions.
7. Remove the needle carefully and immediately dispose of it in the sharps bin.
8. Clean the area with gauze.

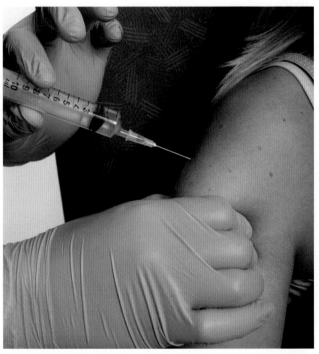

Fig. 4.4 Enter the skin at 90°.

9. Inform the patient to let a member of staff know if the site is painful, bleeds or if they have any other concerns.
10. Remove gloves and wash hands.
11. Document the drug administration in the drug chart.

DOCUMENT THE PROCEDURE

Document under the following headings:
- IM injection given
- Date, time and place
- Indications for the procedure
- Patient consent
- Allergy status
- Site used
- Name and amount of medication given, expiry date and batch number
- Complications

QUESTIONS AND ANSWERS FOR CANDIDATE

Name three medications that can be administered intramuscularly.
- Naloxone
- Methotrexate
- Morphine
- Prednisolone
- Haloperidol
- Testosterone
- Vitamin B$_{12}$
- Cyclizine

Name three complications that you might see with an IM injection.
- Pain
- Bleeding
- Infection
- Injuries to nerves and blood vessels
- Unintentional intravenous access

Mark Scheme for Examiner

	0	1	2	3
Introduction and General Advice				
Introduces self and washes hands				
Confirms patient's identity with three points of identification				
Explains procedure, identifies concerns and obtains consent				
Checks for allergies and needle phobia				
Preparation				
Obtains equipment and checks expiry dates				
Washes hands and dons non-sterile gloves				
Attaches syringe to needle for drawing up medication				
Selects appropriate site for injection				
Cleans injection site				
Checks medication and prescription with colleague				
Draws up medication				
IM Injection				
Changes needle				
Stabilises skin around injection site				
Checks for flashback and then injects medication at 90°				
Disposes of sharps				
Finishing				
Tells patient to inform staff if site becomes painful or continues to bleed				
Signs the patient's drug chart				
Disposes of equipment and cleans tray				
Removes gloves and washes hands				
Washes hands				
General Points				
Talks to the patient throughout the procedure				
Avoids patient contamination (i.e. non-touch technique [NTT])				

0 = Not attempted
1 = Performed, with room for improvement
2 = Adequately performed
3 = Performed beyond level expected

What are the most common muscle groups used for IM injections?

- Vastus lateralis
- Rectus femoris
- Deltoid
- Ventrogluteal

What is a known complication of IM injections into the dorsogluteal muscle?

- Sciatic nerve injury

What factors need to be taken into account when selecting the size/length of the needle?

- Muscle group that the injection is going into
- Patient's weight/body habitus
- Amount of subcutaneous fat

 Tip Box

Many centres will now use safety needles for injections. Usage of each safety needle varies; follow individual instructions.

 Fact Box

IM medications are absorbed quicker than subcutaneous (SC) medications because there is a greater vascular supply to muscle tissues than to the SC tissues. Muscle tissues are also larger in volume.

STATION 4.2: SUBCUTANEOUS INJECTIONS

SCENARIO

Mrs Jin is a new patient on your ward. She requires venous thromboembolism (VTE) prophylaxis. Please administer her prescribed subcutaneous (SC) low-molecular-weight heparin (LMWH).

OBJECTIVE

- Administering SC injections

GENERAL ADVICE

- When administering any injection, remember it is important to ensure that the patient has no known drug allergies, that you obtain verbal consent and that you wear gloves.
- When determining the site for the injections, try to avoid areas showing broken skin, infection, inflammation or swelling.
- If a patient needs daily injections, remember to rotate the injection site to avoid skin irritation, lipohypertrophy, lipoatrophy or lipodystrophy.
- In the palliative care setting, many of the commonly used medications are administered subcutaneously via a syringe driver.

EQUIPMENT CHECKLIST

(Remember to check expiry dates on all equipment [Fig. 4.5].)

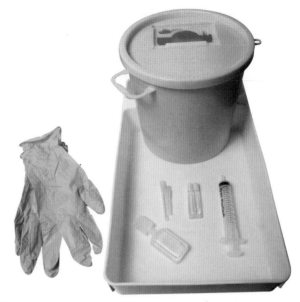

Fig. 4.5 Gather your equipment.

- Tray: Either single-use, disposable sterilised tray, or a decontaminated plastic tray that is cleaned pre-/post-procedure
- Non-sterile gloves
- Skin-cleansing solution
- 25-gauge needle
- 21-gauge needle or filter needle for drawing up medication
- Medication for injection
- Syringe (size depending on injection)
- Sharps bin: The sharps bin should always be taken to the point of care
- Sterile gauze

Note: Skin-cleansing solutions and method will vary depending on local policy.

EXPLAINING SC INJECTION TO THE PATIENT

1. We need to give you some medication under your skin.
2. A small needle connected to a syringe will be inserted just underneath your skin.
3. It will be slightly painful.
4. The syringe contains your medication, which will be injected just under your skin so that it can go into your body system.

PREPARATION FOR ALL INJECTIONS

1. Obtain consent.
2. Wash hands and don a pair of non-sterile gloves.
3. Inspect the proposed site for injection and ensure it is suitable.
4. Clean site following local policy. Allow to dry fully.
5. With a colleague, check the drug dose against the drug chart and check the drug expiry date.
6. Draw up the medication using a syringe and a 21-gauge needle if using a plastic ampoule, or a filter needle if using a glass ampoule.
7. Expel any excess air in the syringe.

SUBCUTANEOUS INJECTION

1. Discard the 21-gauge needle in the sharps bin and replace it with a new 25-gauge needle.
2. Pinch the skin to ensure the adipose tissue is separated from the underlying muscle layer.
3. Hold the syringe like a pencil between your thumb and forefinger.
4. Insert the whole needle into the adipose tissue at 45° or 90° depending on the medication (Fig. 4.6).
5. Slowly inject the medication according to the instructions.
6. Remove the needle carefully and immediately dispose of it in the sharps bin.
7. Clean the area with gauze.
8. Inform the patient to let a member of staff know if the site is painful, bleeds, or if they have any other concerns.
9. Remove gloves and wash hands.

DOCUMENT THE PROCEDURE

Document under the following headings:

- SC injection given
- Date, time and place
- Indications for the procedure
- Patient consent
- Allergy status
- Site used
- Name and amount of medication given, expiry date and batch number
- Complications

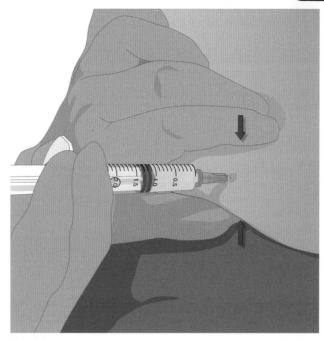

Fig. 4.6 Enter the skin at 45° or 90° depending on the medication being given.

Mark Scheme for Examiner

	0	1	2	3
Introduction and General Advice				
Introduces self and washes hands				
Confirms patient's identity with three points of identification				
Explains procedure, identifies concerns and obtains consent				
Checks for allergies and needle phobia				
Preparation				
Obtains equipment and checks expiry dates				
Washes hands and dons non-sterile gloves				
Attaches syringe to needle for drawing up medication				
Selects appropriate site for injection				
Cleans injection site				
Checks medication and prescription with colleague				
Draws up medication				
SC Injection				
Changes needle				
Pinches skin				
Inserts needle at 45° or 90°				
Disposes of sharps				
Finishing				
Tells patient to inform staff if site becomes painful or continues to bleed				
Signs the patient's drug chart				
Disposes of equipment and cleans tray				
Removes gloves and washes hands				

Continued

Mark Scheme for Examiner—cont'd

	0	1	2	3
General Points				
Talks to the patient throughout the procedure				
Avoids patient contamination (i.e. NTT)				

0 = Not attempted
1 = Performed, with room for improvement
2 = Adequately performed
3 = Performed beyond level expected

QUESTIONS AND ANSWERS FOR CANDIDATE

What signs would indicate that the patient may be experiencing a local allergic reaction to a drug administered by injection?
- Urticarial rash
- Localised swelling
- Pruritus

How would you convert 20 mg of oral (PO) morphine to SC morphine?
- Halve the dose

What scoring criteria can be used to define a patient's risk of developing a deep-vein thrombosis (DVT)?
- Wells score

What prophylactic measures are there to prevent VTE?
- Antiembolic stockings
- Intermittent pneumatic compression
- Pharmacological prophylaxis, e.g. LMWH, unfractionated heparin, fondaparinux

When might you give SC fluids, rather than IV fluids?
- End-of-life care

Tip Box

If you want to practise SC injections, inpatients usually receive their prophylactic LWMH around 6 p.m. so you can hang around the ward until then one evening and ask the nurse if you can kindly join them on their medication round and administer some SC injections.

Fact Box

Common medications that are administered subcutaneously at 90° are LMWH and insulin. Most other medications are injected at 45°.

STATION 4.3: INTRADERMAL INJECTIONS

SCENARIO

Mrs Gupta is a 32-year-old woman attending your dermatology outpatient clinic. She has been referred for allergy testing. Please demonstrate the method of an intradermal injection.

OBJECTIVE

- Administering intradermal injection

GENERAL ADVICE

- When administering any injection, it is important to ensure that the patient has no known drug allergies, that you obtain verbal consent and that you wear gloves.
- When determining the site for the injections, try to avoid areas showing broken skin, infection, inflammation or swelling.

EQUIPMENT CHECKLIST

(Remember to check expiry dates on all equipment [Fig. 4.7].)
- Tray: Either single-use, disposable sterilised tray, or a decontaminated plastic tray that is cleaned pre-/post-procedure
- Non-sterile gloves
- Skin-cleansing solution
- 25-gauge needle
- 21-gauge needle or filter needle for drawing up medication
- Medication for injection
- Syringe (size depending on injection)
- Sharps bin: The sharps bin should always be taken to the point of care
- Sterile gauze

Note: Skin-cleansing solutions and method will vary depending on local policy.

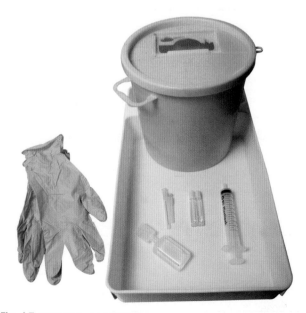

Fig. 4.7 Gather your equipment.

EXPLAINING INTRADERMAL INJECTION TO THE PATIENT

1. We need to give you some medication into your skin.
2. A small needle connected to a syringe will be inserted into one of the layers of your skin.
3. It will be slightly painful.
4. The syringe contains a substance which will be injected into your skin.

PREPARATION FOR ALL INJECTIONS

1. Obtain consent.
2. Wash hands and don a pair of non-sterile gloves.
3. Inspect the proposed site for injection and ensure it is suitable.
4. Clean site following local policy. Allow to dry fully.
5. With a colleague, check the drug dose against the drug chart and check the drug expiry date.
6. Draw up the medication using a syringe and a 21-gauge needle if using a plastic ampoule, or a filter needle if using a glass ampoule.
7. Expel any excess air in the syringe.

INTRADERMAL INJECTION

1. Discard the 21-gauge needle in the sharps bin and replace it with a new 25-gauge needle.
2. Hold the syringe like a pencil between thumb and forefinger.
3. Insert the needle below the epidermis at 10 to 15° with the bevel pointing upward.
4. Slowly inject the medication according to the instructions and watch a bleb form (Fig. 4.8).
5. Remove the needle carefully and immediately dispose of it into the sharps bin.

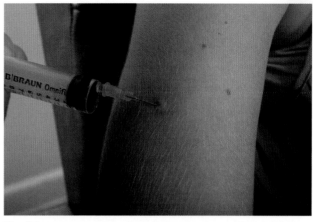

Fig. 4.8 Ensure you form a bleb when giving an intradermal injection.

6. Clean the area with gauze.
7. Inform the patient to let a member of staff know if the site is painful, bleeds, or if they have any other concerns.
8. Remove gloves and wash hands.

DOCUMENT THE PROCEDURE

Document under the following headings:
- Intradermal injection given
- Date, time and place
- Indications for the procedure
- Patient consent
- Allergy status
- Site used
- Name and amount of product(s) given, expiry date and batch number
- Complications

Mark Scheme for Examiner

	0	1	2	3
Introduction and General Advice				
Introduces self and washes hands				
Confirms patient's identity with three points of identification				
Explains procedure, identifies concerns and obtains consent				
Checks for allergies and needle phobia				
Preparation				
Obtains equipment and checks expiry dates				
Washes hands and dons non-sterile gloves				
Attaches syringe to needle for drawing up medication				
Selects appropriate site for injection				
Cleans injection site				
Checks medication and prescription with colleague				
Draws up medication				
Intradermal injection				
Changes needle				
Pinches skin				
Inserts needle at 10–15°				
Disposes of sharps				

Continued

Mark Scheme for Examiner—cont'd

	0	1	2	3
Finishing				
Tells patient to inform staff if site becomes painful or continues to bleed				
Signs the patient's drug chart				
Disposes of equipment and cleans tray				
Removes gloves and washes hands				
General Points				
Talks to the patient throughout the procedure				
Avoids patient contamination (i.e. NTT)				

0 = Not attempted
1 = Performed, with room for improvement
2 = Adequately performed
3 = Performed beyond level expected

❓ QUESTIONS AND ANSWERS FOR CANDIDATE

Which medications commonly interfere with skin allergy testing?
- Antihistamine medication
- Antidepressants

What is the difference between a skin prick test and a skin patch test?
- Skin prick tests are used to diagnose hayfever allergies.
- Skin patch tests are used to find out whether the patient's dermatitis is aggravated by a contact allergy.

What should the patient note when going for a skin patch test?
- Remark the test sites if necessary.
- Keep the testing area dry.
- Do not expose the back to the sun for 4 weeks prior to the patch tests.

What is an 'angry back' in the context of skin patch testing?
- An 'angry back' reaction refers to false positives to many or all of the tested allergens. It occurs more commonly in patients with active dermatitis at the time of testing.

What are the main medications used in the management of anaphylactic shock?
- IM adrenaline
- IM or IV chlorphenamine
- IM or IV hydrocortisone
- Doses vary depending on the patient's age

Tip Box

Some patients feel more comfortable looking away while receiving an injection so present this option to them before you start.

Fact Box

Intradermal injections are commonly used for allergy and tuberculin testing. Due to the location, only small volumes (<2 mL) are used. These are usually performed on the inner aspect of the forearm or the upper back.

STATION 4.4: LOCAL ANAESTHETIC ADMINISTRATION

SCENARIO

Miss Page is a 24-year-old woman who is suffering with a headache, nausea and double vision. Her neurologist would like a lumbar puncture (LP) to be performed. You are asked to insert the local anaesthetic (LA) before your registrar completes the LP.

OBJECTIVE

- Learning how to administer LA

GENERAL ADVICE

- Introduce yourself.
- Explain what injection LA involves: This should include the fact that the patient will experience some pain from the initial injection and that LA does sting when it is injected.
- Obtain verbal consent.
- Check for the patient's allergies.
- Make sure you know the area into which you will inject the LA for the specific procedure and that the skin is not damaged, broken or inflamed.
- Depending on the procedure, the infiltration of the LA will differ, i.e. it will be superficial for a skin biopsy but deeper for procedures such as an LP or therapeutic paracentesis.

EQUIPMENT CHECKLIST

(Remember to check expiry dates on all equipment.)
- Tray: Either single-use, disposable sterilised tray, or a decontaminated plastic tray that is cleaned pre-/post-procedure
- Non-sterile gloves
- Skin-cleansing solution
- 21–25-gauge needle(s)
- 21-gauge needle or filter needle for drawing up medication
- Medication for injection
- Syringe (size depending on injection)

- Sharps bin: The sharps bin should always be taken to the point of care

Note: Skin-cleansing solutions and method will vary depending on local policy.

EXPLAINING LA INJECTION TO THE PATIENT

1. We need to give you some medication through your skin that will numb the area so that you don't feel any pain during the procedure.
2. A small needle connected to a syringe will be inserted and this syringe contains a local anaesthetic agent that will be injected.
3. You will feel a bit of pain at the beginning as the initial injection is made but then it should start to ease, and you'll only feel the pressure of the instruments, not any pain.

PREPARATION FOR ALL INJECTIONS

1. Obtain consent.
2. Wash hands and don a pair of non-sterile gloves.
3. Inspect the proposed site for injection and ensure it is suitable.
4. Clean site following local policy. Allow to dry fully.
5. With a colleague, check the drug dose against the drug chart and check the drug expiry date.
6. Draw up the medication using a syringe and a 21-gauge needle if using a plastic ampoule, or a filter needle if using a glass ampoule.
7. Expel any excess air in the syringe.

LOCAL ANAESTHETIC INJECTION

1. Discard the 21-gauge needle in the sharps bin and replace it with a new 25-gauge needle.
2. Hold the syringe like a pencil between thumb and forefinger.
3. Insert the needle at 10–15° into the taut injection site and slowly infiltrate until you see bleb formation (Refer to Fig. 4.8).
4. Then, if required, change the 25-gauge needle to a 21-gauge needle for deeper infiltration, insert the needle through the anaesthetised skin and draw back in the syringe for 5 s to check that the needle has not penetrated a vein (Fig. 4.9).

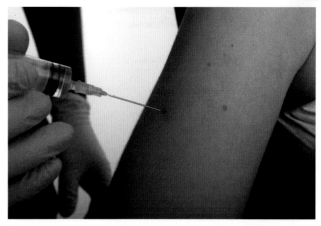

Fig. 4.9 If required, reposition the needle for deeper infiltration.

5. If there is no flashback, then proceed. If there is flashback, withdraw the needle slightly and recheck for flashback.
6. Slowly infiltrate the anaesthetic at a rate in accordance with the instructions. The depth and amount of LA given will depend on the specific procedure.
7. Remove the needle carefully and immediately dispose of it in the sharps bin.
8. Wait a few minutes before starting the procedure and always check that the skin is anaesthetised before beginning.
9. At the end of the procedure, inform the patient to let a member of staff know if the site is painful, bleeds, or if they have any other concerns.
10. Remove gloves and wash hands.
11. Document the drug administration in the drug chart.

DOCUMENT THE PROCEDURE

Document under the following headings:
- LA injection given
- Date, time and place
- Indications for the procedure
- Patient consent
- Allergy status
- Site used
- Name and amount of LA given, expiry date and batch number
- Complications

🔲 Mark Scheme for Examiner

	0	1	2	3
Introduction and General Advice				
Introduces self and washes hands				
Confirms patient's identity with three points of identification				
Explains procedure, identifies concerns and obtains consent				
Checks for allergies and needle phobia				
Preparation				
Obtains equipment and checks expiry dates				
Washes hands and dons non-sterile gloves				

Continued

Mark Scheme for Examiner—cont'd

	0	1	2	3
Attaches syringe to needle for drawing up medication				
Selects appropriate site for injection				
Cleans injection site				
Checks medication and prescription with colleague				
Draws up medication				
LA Injection				
Checks for flashback before injecting				
Begins with an intradermal bleb at 15° under the skin and checks response				
Administers appropriate amount of LA to the correct depth for the specific procedure				
Waits for the LA to take effect before continuing with specific procedure				
Disposes of sharps				
Finishing				
Tells patient to inform staff if site becomes painful or continues to bleed				
Signs the patient's drug chart				
Disposes of equipment and cleans tray				
Removes gloves and washes hands				
General Points				
Talks to the patient throughout the procedure				
Avoids patient contamination (i.e. NTT)				

0 = Not attempted
1 = Performed, with room for improvement
2 = Adequately performed
3 = Performed beyond level expected

❓ QUESTIONS AND ANSWERS FOR CANDIDATE

Why is LA sometimes used with adrenaline?
- The adrenaline stops the LA from being rapidly redistributed by the circulation and therefore its action is enhanced at the required area. Adrenaline must be used with caution in the extremities due to the potential risk of ischaemia.

What are the two basic classes of LA?
- Amino amides
- Amino esters

Name three examples of LA.
- Bupivacaine
- Levobupivacaine
- Lidocaine
- Prilocaine
- Ropivacaine
- Tetracaine

What is LA toxicity, and when does it occur?
- An adverse reaction from administration of a high volume of LA, leading to events of acute neurotoxicity and cardiac toxicity
- LA toxicity typically manifests in minutes, up to 1 h, after the initial administration

How do you manage LA toxicity?
- Stop injection of LA.
- Symptomatic management, e.g. control seizures, treat hypotension, bradycardia and arrhythmias.
- If the patient is in circulatory arrest, start cardiopulmonary resuscitation.
- Consider giving IV lipid emulsion in accordance with the guidelines.

 Tip Box

Remember that after the first injection, subsequent injections through the infiltrated area are less painful.

 Fact Box

LA is effective for approximately 4 to 6 h, but the duration can vary depending on the type of anaesthetic used.

STATION 4.5: INTRAVENOUS DRUGS

SCENARIO

You are the junior doctor on the ward. One of your post-operative patients, Mrs Chi, has become unwell overnight, spiking temperatures and requires IV antibiotics. Please discuss with your examiner how you would give the antibiotics.

OBJECTIVE

- Administering IV medication

GENERAL ADVICE

- When administering IV medication, it is important that you are familiar with the therapeutic use of the drug and the possible side effects.
- Ensure that the patient has no known drug allergies, that you obtain verbal consent and that you wear gloves.
- Check the prescription and if you have any concerns, check with the prescriber.

EQUIPMENT CHECKLIST

(Remember to check expiry dates on all equipment.)
- Tray: Either single-use, disposable sterilised tray, or a decontaminated plastic tray that is cleaned pre-/post-procedure
- Non-sterile gloves
- Skin-cleansing solution
- Prescribed IV drug
- 10 mL 0.9% saline for flush
- Giving set (if required)
- Two 21-gauge needles (or filter needles)
- 10-mL syringe (size depending on injection)
- Sharps bin: The sharps bin should always be taken to the point of care

Note: Skin-cleansing solutions and method will vary depending on local policy.

EXPLAINING IV INJECTION TO THE PATIENT

1. We need to give you some medication through your veins.
2. We will connect the medication to the cannula that you already have, and it will automatically go into your veins.
3. It should not cause any pain, but you might feel the medication running up through your arms initially.

ADMINISTERING IV MEDICATION

CHECKS AND PREPARATION

1. Introduce yourself to the patient and obtain consent.
2. Check the patient's name, hospital number and date of birth.
3. Check the prescriber's signature.
4. Check the prescription dose, date, time and route of admission.
5. Check the patient's allergy status.
6. Check the batch number and expiry date of the medication and flush.
7. Check medication for discoloration or cloudiness.
8. Check that the patient has a patent IV cannula in situ.
9. Check that the cannula site has no sign of infection or phlebitis.
10. Collect the equipment you require.
11. Wash hands and don non-sterile gloves.

GIVING AN IV INJECTION

1. Clean the coloured port of the cannula using skin-cleansing solution.
2. Check the cannula is patent by flushing (assembled as previously described) 5 mL of 0.9% saline through the port (Fig. 4.10).
3. Tap the medication ampoule to dislodge any medication at the neck and snap open.
4. Draw up the correct volume of medication using a needle and syringe:
   - If the medication is in a glass vial, use a filter needle to draw up the medication to avoid aspiration of glass shards.
   - If the medication is in a powder, reconstitute the solution following the manufacturer's guidelines.
5. Tap the syringe to dislodge any air bubbles to the top of the syringe. Immediately dispose of any sharps.
6. Expel any air that is left in the syringe and dispose of the needle in the sharps bin.
7. Attach the syringe to the cannula and administer the IV medication as directed by the drug manufacturer's guidelines.
8. Flush the cannula with the remaining 5 mL of 0.9% saline.
9. Check the cannula site.

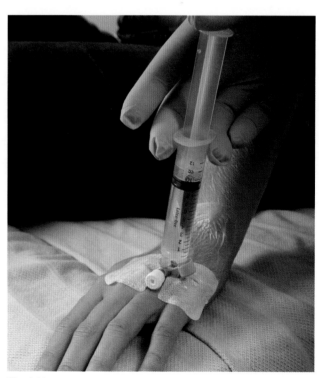

Fig. 4.10 Always flush with 0.9% saline.

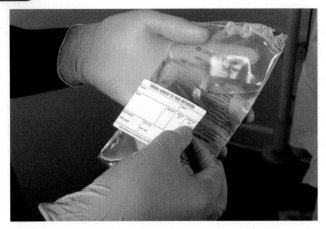

Fig. 4.11 An example of an additive label.

GIVING AN IV INFUSION

1. Complete an IV additive label (available from the pharmacy) and attach it to the fluid bag (Fig. 4.11). The label must state:
   - Patient's name, hospital number and date of birth
   - Name, dose and batch number of the medication
   - Expiry date of the medication
   - Date and time the medication was added to the bag
   - Signatures of the healthcare professionals administering and checking the medication
2. Clean the injection port on the fluid bag with skin-cleansing solution.
3. Inject the medication into the fluid bag via the injection port.

4. Dispose of sharps.
5. Gently turn the fluid bag upside down several times to mix the drug with the fluid. Clean the cannula port.
6. Follow the instructions as outlined in station 3.7 (to prepare the fluid and giving set). Once completed, hang the IV fluid bag up on a drip stand and allow the fluid to run through into the cannula.
7. Hang the IV fluid bag and calculate the flow rate as directed by the prescription.

FINISHING

1. Sign the drug chart, stating the date and time when the medication was given.
2. Monitor the patient's observations to ensure that there is no acute reaction.

DOCUMENT THE PROCEDURE

Document under the following headings:
- IV injection given
- Date, time and place
- Indications for the procedure
- Patient consent
- Allergy status
- Cannula used
- Name and amount of medication given, expiry date and batch number
- Time medication was started/given
- Complications

Mark Scheme for Examiner

	0	1	2	3
Introduction and General Advice				
Introduces self and washes hands				
Confirms patient's identity with three points of identification				
Explains procedure, identifies concerns and obtains consent				
Checks for allergies				
Preparation				
Obtains equipment and checks expiry dates				
Washes hands and dons non-sterile gloves				
Attaches syringe to needle for drawing up medication				
Checks prescription				
Checks medication and flush				
Checks cannula site				
IV Injection				
Draws up flush and checks cannula patency				
Checks cannula patency				
Opens ampoule and draws up medication				
Expels air				
Gives medication through cannula				
Flushes cannula				

Continued

📖 Mark Scheme for Examiner—cont'd

	0	1	2	3
Checks cannula site				
IV Infusion				
Completes IV additive label				
Cleans injection port				
Injects medication into fluid bag. Disposes of sharps				
Mixes medication and fluid				
Cleans cannula port				
Sets up the IV giving set				
Calculates the drip rate				
Finishing				
Signs the patient's drug chart				
Disposes of equipment and cleans tray				
Removes gloves and washes hands				
Assesses patient to ensure no acute drug reaction				
General Points				
Talks to the patient throughout the procedure				
Avoids patient contamination (i.e. NTT)				

0 = Not attempted
1 = Performed, with room for improvement
2 = Adequately performed
3 = Performed beyond level expected

❓ QUESTIONS AND ANSWERS FOR CANDIDATE

What are the possible complications of IV administration of medication?
- Phlebitis
- Extravasion into soft tissue
- Air embolism
- Drug reaction

What are the advantages of giving a drug IV?
- Immediate delivery of medication into the blood stream
- Precise quantity of drug delivered into the blood stream

What are the disadvantages of giving a drug IV?
- Requires the patient to have IV access
- Risks associated with cannulation

Which drugs are particularly irritable to the skin and could cause extravasation?
- Chemotherapy medications
- Phenytoin
- Noradrenaline
- 50% glucose

Which patients are more at risk of extravasation injuries?
- Patients who have difficulty with communication
- Children
- Patients with reduced Glasgow Coma Scale
- Patients with fragile or thin skin
- Patients with peripheral neuropathy

 Tip Box

Ensure you follow Trust policy for checking IV medication. Usually it should be checked by two qualified healthcare professionals to ensure patient safety.

 Fact Box

Extravasation injury is the inadvertent leakage of a vesicant solution, whereas infiltration is the inadvertent leakage of a non-vesicant solution.

STATION 4.6: DRUG ADMINISTRATION VIA NEBULISER

SCENARIO

Mr Netherby is a 49-year-old man with known chronic asthma. He has presented to hospital with shortness of breath, inability to speak in full sentences, tachycardia and tachypnoea. You have been asked to give Mr Netherby salbutamol via a nebuliser.

OBJECTIVES

- Learning the indications for administering nebulised medication
- Administering medication via a nebuliser

GENERAL ADVICE

- When administering any medication, it is important to ensure:
  - The patient has no known drug allergies
  - That you gain verbal consent
  - That you wear gloves

EQUIPMENT CHECKLIST

(Remember to check expiry dates on all equipment.)
- Tray: Either single-use, disposable sterilised tray, or a decontaminated plastic tray that is cleaned pre-/post-procedure
- Non-sterile gloves
- Oxygen mask (check the prescription chart for which mask should be used)
- Oxygen tubing
- 10-mL syringe (to draw up medication. Requires additional equipment for preparing medication depending on specific drug, e.g. 0.9% saline)
- Prescribed oxygen
- Prescribed medication

EXPLAINING GIVING DRUGS VIA A NEBULISER TO THE PATIENT

1. We need to give you some medication through a mask that you wear over your face. This mask is called a nebuliser.
2. We will pour the medication that you need into the nebuliser.
3. Then you will wear this mask over your mouth and nose, and it will drive the medication into your lungs as you breathe normally.
4. It should not cause any pain.

DRUG ADMINISTRATION VIA NEBULISER

1. Wash hands and don a pair of non-sterile gloves.
2. Position the patient upright, if possible.
3. Check the expiry date of the medication.
4. Draw up the prescribed medication into a sterile syringe. Place the medication into the nebuliser. Note whether the patient is to have the medication through oxygen or just air. If oxygen is prescribed, connect the nebuliser to oxygen tubing.
5. Ensure that mist is being released from the mask, indicating that the nebuliser is working.

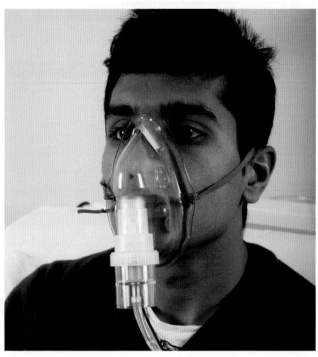

Fig. 4.12 Ensure you are familiar with the nebulisers used in your trust.

6. Apply the face mask to the patient. Instruct the patient to breathe normally through the mouth (Fig. 4.12).
7. Dispose of the syringe.
8. Document the drug administration in the drug chart.
9. Assess the patient for adverse effects to the medication.
10. Ensure mask and chamber are rinsed and air-dried after each use.

DOCUMENT THE PROCEDURE

Document under the following headings:
- Nebuliser given
- Date, time and place
- Indications for the procedure
- Patient consent
- Allergy status
- Name and amount of medication given, expiry date and batch number
- Time medication was started/given
- Complications

Mark Scheme for Examiner

	0	1	2	3
Introduction and General Advice				
Introduces self and washes hands				
Confirms patient's identity with three points of identification				
Explains procedure, identifies concerns and obtains consent				
Checks for allergies				
Preparation				
Obtains equipment and checks expiry dates				
Washes hands and dons non-sterile gloves				
Positions the patient upright				
Administering Medication				
Draws up medication				
Places medication in the nebuliser				
Connects face mask, nebuliser and oxygen				
Applies face mask and asks the patient to breathe normally				
Finishing				
Monitors the patient				
Signs the patient's drug chart				
Disposes of equipment and cleans tray				
Removes gloves and washes hands				
General Points				
Talks to the patient throughout the procedure				
Avoids patient contamination (i.e. NTT)				

0 = Not attempted
1 = Performed, with room for improvement
2 = Adequately performed
3 = Performed beyond level expected

❓ QUESTIONS AND ANSWERS FOR CANDIDATE

Name three medications that might be administered via a nebuliser.
- β-agonists
- Mucolytics
- Anticholinergics
- Antibiotics
- Antimicrobials (for example, pentamidine for pneumocystis pneumonia)
- Adrenaline

How should nebulisers be maintained and cleaned?
- Ideally nebulisers should be washed after each use.
- The mask, mouthpiece and chamber should be disconnected and then individually washed in warm, soapy water. Leave them to air dry on a clean tissue or kitchen paper towel before next use.

How many times would a patient be using his reliever inhaler before you consider stepping up his asthma management plan?
- At least three times per week

Can patients have nebulisers at home?
- Yes, but this is usually recommended by their respiratory team and the patient will need to be appropriately trained.

Name three triggers that could potentially cause an asthma exacerbation.
- Infections
- Physical exercise
- Cold temperature
- Dry or polluted air, including chemical fumes, smoke or strong odours
- Exposure to allergens, e.g. pets, moulds, grass, pollen, dust mites

 Tip Box

In the majority of patients in an acute setting, it is best to use a non-rebreather mask if the type of oxygen mask has not been specified on the oxygen prescription chart. Do note, however, that in some patients, such as those with chronic obstructive pulmonary disease (COPD), you may need to control the amount of oxygen delivered with the nebuliser accurately. This can be achieved using a Venturi mask.

 Fact Box

A clinician may choose to prescribe salbutamol nebuliser rather than inhalers because oxygen needs to be given at the same time. Otherwise, inhalers are equally effective.

STATION 4.7: OPERATING A SYRINGE DRIVER

SCENARIO

Mrs Peach is a 79-year-old woman who has known metastatic breast cancer. She has been admitted to hospital with pneumonia and uncontrolled pain. She has been deteriorating and is now unable to swallow tablets. The patient, along with her family and the medical team, have made a decision that she will receive supportive care only. Please discuss the use of syringe drivers with the examiner.

OBJECTIVES

- To know the indications for commencing a syringe driver
- To understand the general principles of operating a syringe driver

GENERAL ADVICE

There are currently many different types of syringe drivers used in hospitals. Ensure that you familiarise yourself and have training with the particular model used in your trust. Some automatically calculate the infusion rates whilst others require the infusion rate to be set manually (Fig. 4.13).
- When drawing up medication for a syringe driver, the drugs should be checked by two members of the nursing/medical staff using the prescription chart.
- Some trusts permit single-nurse administration as long as no controlled drugs are used.
- Each syringe used should be labelled with the patient's name, date of birth, the names and doses of drugs, diluent, total volume, time, date and signatures of those preparing the medication.
- Each syringe should carry enough medication for 24 h.

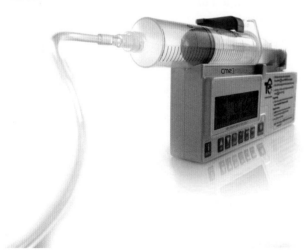

Fig. 4.13 T34 ambulatory syringe pump. Common component parts are found in all syringe drivers, but ensure you are familiar with those used in your trust. (Courtesy of CME Medical UK Ltd)

- Syringe drivers are locked inside a plastic cage to ensure that they cannot be tampered with. The nurse in charge usually holds the key to the cage.
- Most syringe drivers are battery-powered and the batteries can often be changed whilst the driver is locked inside the plastic cage.

INSERTING THE METAL NEEDLE OR PLASTIC CANNULA

There are different types of giving sets in use. Metal needles are more commonly found in hospitals and the community, whereas plastic cannulae are more commonly found in hospices.

EQUIPMENT CHECKLIST

(Remember to check expiry dates on all equipment.)
- Tray: Either single-use, disposable sterilised tray, or a decontaminated plastic tray that is cleaned pre-/post-procedure
- Two pairs of non-sterile gloves
- Skin-cleansing solution
- Metal needle or cannula
- Infusion line and giving set
- Syringe driver
- Battery
- Medication in labelled syringe
- Clear film dressing
- Lockable box (if used)
- Carry case (if used)

EXPLAINING A SYRINGE DRIVER TO THE PATIENT

1. A syringe driver is a small portable pump that supplies medication continuously via a line attached to a syringe.
2. Syringe drivers are useful when patients find tablets hard to swallow. Instead, a small needle or plastic tube is placed just underneath your skin, which allows the medication to enter the body.
3. Several different drugs can be put through the syringe driver to help with symptoms such as pain, nausea and vomiting.
4. Medication is supplied throughout the 24-h period, helping to control symptoms consistently, as the amount of each drug in the blood stream should remain constant.
5. Although the skin at the site of the needle can get wet, the pump itself should be kept dry.

SETTING UP THE SYRINGE DRIVER

1. Obtain consent.
2. Wash hands and put on non-sterile gloves.
3. Make up the medication solution as prescribed in an appropriately sized syringe.

4. Prime the line and giving set in accordance with manufacturers' instructions, and attach the syringe to the syringe driver.
5. Confirm patient identity in accordance with Trust policy.
6. Locate an insertion site. The giving set can be inserted subcutaneously in a site with adipose tissue, providing it is not inflamed or oedematous. Avoid using areas where radiotherapy is targeted. The site of insertion should be checked at least once a day for inflammation, soreness, hardening of the skin or infection. If any of these are seen, the site should be changed immediately. Sites used commonly are:
   • Upper arm
   • Abdomen
   • Chest
   • Thigh
7. Wash your hands and put on a new pair of non-sterile gloves.
8. Clean the area of insertion using skin-cleansing solution.
9. Insert the needle or cannula into the skin at an angle of 45° and cover with clear film dressing to secure in place.
10. Set the pump to run at the correct rate.
11. Put the pump in a lockable box or carry case (if used).
12. Remove gloves and wash hands.
13. Document the date, time, rate of infusion, battery status and insertion site in the patient's notes.
14. Sign the patient's drug chart.

Drugs Commonly Used in Syringe Drivers for Palliation

Drug	Indications	Important information
Cyclizine	Nausea Vomiting	Can cause insertion site inflammation. This can be helped by diluting the drug well with 'water for injection'
Dexamethasone	Antiemetic Pain Raised intracranial pressure	Advisable to put in a separate syringe driver in larger doses instead of mixing it with another drug
Diamorphine	Pain Shortness of breath Cough	Mixes well with most drugs
Haloperidol	Nausea Vomiting Hiccups	Extrapyramidal side effects can occur with high doses
Hyoscine hydrobromide	Excess secretion	Mixes well with most drugs
Metoclopramide	Nausea Vomiting Delayed gastric emptying	Mixes well with most drugs
Midazolam	Agitation Epilepsy Muscle spasm	Mixes well with most drugs

Mark Scheme for Examiner

	0	1	2	3
Introduction and General Advice				
Introduces self and washes hands				
Confirms patient's identity with three points of identification				
Explains procedure, identifies concerns and obtains consent				
Checks for allergies				
Setting Up the Syringe Driver				
Obtains equipment, medication and checks expiry dates				
Washes hands and dons non-sterile gloves				
Makes up medication in appropriately sized syringe. Labels each syringe correctly				
Primes the line and giving set with the medication				
Attaches syringe to syringe driver				

Continued

Mark Scheme for Examiner—cont'd

	0	1	2	3
Inserting the Metal Needle or Plastic Cannula				
Locates appropriate site for insertion				
Washes hands, dons non-sterile gloves and cleans insertion site				
Inserts the needle or cannula				
Sets rate on syringe driver				
Covers needle/cannula with clear dressing				
Finishing				
Tells patient to inform staff if they feel unwell or have any problems with the insertion site				
Signs the patient's drug chart				
Disposes of equipment and cleans tray				
Removes gloves and washes hands				
General Points				
Talks to the patient throughout the procedure				
Avoids patient contamination (i.e. NTT)				

0 = Not attempted
1 = Performed, with room for improvement
2 = Adequately performed
3 = Performed beyond level expected

QUESTIONS AND ANSWERS FOR CANDIDATE

What are some indications for syringe driver use?
- Patients with nausea or vomiting
- Patients with dysphagia
- Patients who are too weak to swallow tablets
- Patients with oral tumours or infections
- Unconscious patients
- Poor patient compliance with other mechanisms of drug administration
- Poor alimentary absorption
- Patients with no intravenous access

What are you looking for when assessing the insertion site of a syringe driver?
- Metal needle or plastic cannula in situ
- Erythema
- Swelling
- Warmth
- Pain or tenderness

What are the advantages of using a syringe driver rather than injections?
- Can control multiple symptoms with one device
- Maintains a constant level of medication
- Avoids repetitive injection administration

Why might you give hyoscine hydrobromide?
- To reduce the amount of secretion

What medications can be used to help with agitation for patients at the end of their lives?
- Haloperidol
- Midazolam

 Tip Box

If you have any worries or concerns regarding syringe drivers, the hospital palliative care team members are usually available for advice. If the prescription for the syringe driver changes, the original syringe should be discarded and a new syringe and infusion line of medication prepared.

Fact Box

Although water is usually recommended to dilute medication, 0.9% saline must be used with diclofenac, ketorolac and ketamine.

Medicine and Surgery

Outline

STATION 5.1: SIMPLE DRESSING CHANGE

SCENARIO

Mrs Clifton is a 62-year-old woman who is under your care following a laparotomy. It has been 2 days since her operation. Please change her abdominal dressing.

OBJECTIVES

- Undertake a simple dressing change

GENERAL ADVICE

- Simple dressing changes are sterile procedures.
- The type of dressing required depends on the nature and size of the wound.
- Most wounds are documented in the nursing notes. Ensure you are familiar with your Trust's policy on documenting wounds and wound management.
- Clinical photography is useful to document wounds.

EQUIPMENT CHECKLIST

(Remember to check expiry dates on all equipment (Fig. 5.1).)
- Tray: either single-use, disposable sterilised tray, or a decontaminated plastic tray that is cleaned pre-/post-procedure
- Two pairs of non-sterile gloves
- Single-use apron
- Gauze
- Sterile water or saline
- Universal sterile container
- Sterile scissors
- Tape

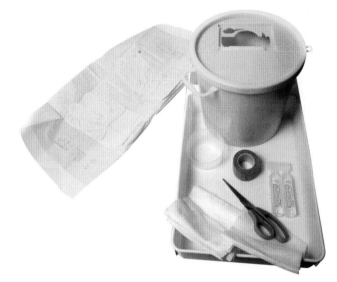

Fig. 5.1 This is a sterile procedure so ensure you have all the equipment you require before going to the patient.

- Surgical dressing
- Clinical waste bag
- Optional: prescribed topical agent, Steri-Strips

SIMPLE DRESSING CHANGE

PREPARATION

1. Introduce yourself to the patient and obtain verbal consent.
2. Adequately expose the wound area.
3. Place the clinical waste bag within reach.
4. Apply single-use apron.
5. Wash hands, and don sterile gloves.
6. Prepare items required for dressing change:
   - Open any packaging.
   - Cut dressings to size using sterile scissors (Fig. 5.2).

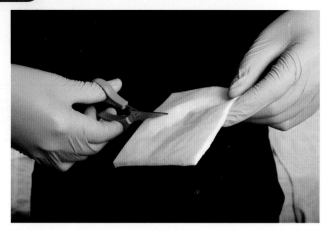

Fig. 5.2 Cut using sterile scissors.

- Cut tape to size.
- Pour sterile water or 0.9% saline into universal container.
- Place initials and date on the dressing or tape.
7. Remove the old dressing and place it in the clinical waste bag.

ASSESSING WOUND

1. Assess the wound:
- Size
- Colour
- Surrounding erythema
- Temperature
- Odour
- Discharge

2. Compare your findings with those documented in the notes.
3. Document your findings in the patient's notes.

CHANGING THE DRESSING

1. Wash hands, and don sterile gloves.
2. Clean the wound with sterile water or normal saline using a washout technique.
3. Pat the skin surrounding the wound dry with gauze.
4. If any cream or ointment has be prescribed, apply using clean gauze as per drug chart.
5. Cover the wound with a new surgical dressing.
6. Remove gloves and place all soiled items into the clinical waste bag.
7. Document the dressing change in the patient's notes.

Summary of Dressings

Dressing	Indication for Use
Film dressing	• Primary dressing • Secondary dressing • Protection from friction or shearing force
Absorbent dressing	• Wound with exudates
Moist dressing	• Dry wound with slough • Necrotic wound
Non-adherent dressing	• Wound with new granulation tissues
Simple island dressing	• Wound with sutures

Mark Scheme for Examiner

	0	1	2	3
Introduction and General Advice				
Introduces self, and washes hands				
Confirms patient's identity with three points of identification				
Explains procedure, identifies concerns and obtains consent				
Checks for allergies if giving medication				
Preparation				
Obtains equipment and checks expiry dates				
Applies single-use apron				
Washes hands, and puts on non-sterile gloves				
Prepares equipment				
Exposes wound by removing old dressing				
Ensures the dressing is the correct size				
Assessing the Wound				
Comments on: size, colour, erythema, temperature, odour, discharge				
Compares findings with those previously documented				
Documents findings				
Dressing Change				
Washes hands, and dons new pair of gloves				
Cleans the wound				
Dries surrounding skin and applies any medications				
Applies new dressing				

Continued

Mark Scheme for Examiner—cont'd

	0	1	2	3
Finishing				
Tells patient to inform staff if wound becomes painful				
Disposes of equipment and cleans tray				
Removes gloves and washes hands				
General Points				
Talks to the patient throughout the procedure				
Avoids patient contamination (i.e. non-touch technique (NTT))				

0= Not attempted
1= Performed, with room for improvement
2= Adequately performed
3= Performed beyond level expected

❓ QUESTIONS AND ANSWERS FOR CANDIDATE

Name three signs of a wound infection.
- Slow healing
- Erythema
- Increasing pain
- Discharge
- Swelling
- Pyrexia

Name three factors that can negatively affect wound healing.
- Age
- Stress
- Diabetes
- Medication; for example, steroids
- Obesity
- Smoking
- Poor nutrition
- Infection
- Inflammation
- Ischaemia

What is the difference between a primary and secondary dressing?
- A primary dressing is one that is placed directly on a wound
- A secondary dressing is one that is used to hold a primary dressing in place

When is a tetanus injection indicated?
- If the patient has had an injury where skin is broken, and the patient's tetanus vaccinations are not up to date

What is the difference between primary- and secondary-intention healing?
- Healing by primary intention occurs when the wound can heal with its dermal edges close together. This usually leads to less scarring and a complete return to function compared to healing by secondary intention.
- Secondary intention healing occurs when the sides of the wounds are not close together, therefore healing must occur from the base of the wound upwards. This increases the chance of scarring.

💡 Tip Box

If the dressing seems stuck when you attempt to remove it from the patient, try moistening the edges with sterile water or 0.9% saline to ease removal.

Fact Box

If there are any new changes to the wound, such as discharge or odour, this may indicate an infection. It is important to swab such wounds and alert the patient's medical team.

STATION 5.2: SPIROMETRY

SCENARIO

Mrs Melini is a 55-year-old woman with a 30-pack-year smoking history. She has come to your clinic complaining of a recurrent productive cough and breathlessness. Perform spirometry, and interpret the results.

OBJECTIVES

- Learn how to perform spirometry
- Measure the forced expiratory volume in 1 s (FEV_1) and forced vital capacity (FVC), and interpret their results

GENERAL ADVICE

- Ensure that you have introduced yourself, identified the patient and washed your hands.

EQUIPMENT CHECKLIST (FIG. 5.3)

- Spirometer
- Disposable mouthpiece

EXPLAINING SPIROMETRY TO THE PATIENT

1. The spirometer is a machine that measures how well your lungs are working.

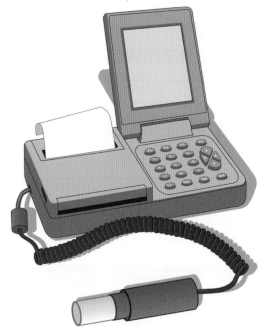

Fig. 5.3 Spirometer and mouthpiece.

2. It gives information such as whether your lungs are expanding sufficiently or whether your airways are narrowed, thereby causing an obstruction to the flow of air out of the lungs.

3. I will demonstrate how to use the spirometer first, and then you can have a couple of practise attempts before the readings are actually taken.

4. If you feel faint or light-headed, just stop and breathe normally.

PERFORMING SPIROMETRY

1. Ask the patient to relax and sit up straight.
2. Attach a clean mouthpiece to the spirometer.
3. Ask the patient to breathe in as deeply as they can.
4. Instruct the patient to breathe out as hard and as fast as possible, until their lungs are empty.
5. Repeat the procedure two more times.
6. Document your findings.

DOCUMENT THE PROCEDURE

Document under the following headings:
- Spirometry performed
- Date, time and place
- Indications for the procedure
- Patient consent
- Results

Present Your Findings

Mrs Melini is a 55-year-old woman complaining of a recurrent cough and shortness of breath. Spirometry reveals that she has an FEV_1 of 75% of her predicted value and an FEV_1:FVC ratio of 0.65. This is in keeping with a mild obstructive disorder. Given the nature of her symptoms and her heavy smoking, this is most likely to be chronic obstructive pulmonary disease.

Mark Scheme for Examiner

	0	1	2	3
Introduction and General Advice				
Introduces self, and washes hands				
Confirms patient's identity with three points of identification				
Explains procedure, identifies concerns and obtains consent				
Explaining Spirometry				
Describes the technique of using the spirometer (breathe deeply, then breathe out as hard and fast as possible into the mouthpiece until lungs are empty)				
Mentions it should be done 3 times				
Records the patient's age, sex and height				
Finishing the Consultation				
Elicits patient concerns and questions				
Arranges a follow-up appointment if necessary or offers contact details				
Thanks the patient and closes the consultation				
General Points				
Checks patient understanding throughout the consultation, avoiding medical jargon, and offers information leaflets				
Is polite and engaging with the patient				

0= Not attempted
1= Performed, with room for improvement
2= Adequately performed
3= Performed beyond level expected

❓ QUESTIONS AND ANSWERS FOR CANDIDATE

Give some reasons for inconsistent readings during spirometry.
- Inadequate or incomplete inhalation
- Lips not tight around the mouthpiece
- Exhalation stops before complete expiration
- Coughing

How is the severity of airflow obstruction graded?
- Mild obstruction − FEV_1 between 50% and 80%
- Moderate obstruction − FEV_1 between 30% and 49%
- Severe obstruction − FEV_1 <30% predicted

What factors are considered when calculating an individual's 'normal' spirometry measurement ranges?
- Age
- Height
- Sex
- Ethnicity (although this is controversial, with an unclear physiological basis)

What is a bronchodilator responsiveness test?
- Also known as a reversibility test
- Spirometry is performed before and after a patient inhales a bronchodilator medication; for example, salbutamol

List five causes of restrictive lung disease.
- Interstitial lung disease, e.g. idiopathic pulmonary fibrosis
- Sarcoidosis
- Obesity, including obesity hypoventilation syndrome
- Scoliosis
- Neuromuscular disease

 Tip Box

There are many different spirometers on the market. Ensure you are familiar with the one you are about to use. Some patients may feel light-headed whilst performing spirometry. It is therefore recommended that the patient is seated during the procedure.

 Fact Box

You can distinguish further between different causes of lung disease with abnormal spirometry using a formal set of pulmonary function tests. It is most commonly used to help investigate restrictive-pattern spirometry. One of the most important pieces of information gathered from these tests is the measurement of the diffusion capacity of the lung. This looks at how readily oxygen can diffuse from the alveoli to the blood by measuring the difference between inspired and expired carbon monoxide. It is represented as 'DLCO' (diffusion capacity of the lung for carbon monoxide) or 'TLCO' (transfer factor of the lung for carbon monoxide). It is decreased in any condition that affects the effective alveolar surface area (Table 5.1).

 Table 5.1 Causes of Decreased and Increased DLCO

CAUSES DECREASED DLCO	CAUSES INCREASED DLCO
Interstitial lung disease	Polycythaemia
Pneumonitis	Pulmonary haemorrhage
Sarcoidosis	Left-to-right intracardiac shunt
Asbestosis	Morbid obesity
Miliary tuberculosis	
Heart failure	

STATION 5.3: KNEE JOINT ASPIRATION

SCENARIO

Mr Jenner is a 62-year-old man who presented to hospital with an acutely swollen left knee. On examination, he is pyrexial and his knee is tender, swollen and erythematous with reduced movement. This is the first time the patient has had any trouble with any of his joints. Please perform a diagnostic aspiration of his knee joint.

OBJECTIVE

- Perform a knee joint aspiration

GENERAL ADVICE

- Ensure that your patient has given verbal consent for the procedure.
- It is vital to check whether the patient has any known drug allergies to anaesthetic agents or bleeding disorders as it may be necessary to modify their medication prior to the procedure.

EQUIPMENT CHECKLIST

(Remember to check expiry dates on all equipment (Fig. 5.4).)
- Tray: either single-use, disposable sterilised tray, or a decontaminated plastic tray that is cleaned pre-/post-procedure
- Antiseptic solution
- Sterile universal container
- Sterile gloves
- Single-use apron
- 10-mL syringe
- 25-gauge needle and two 21-gauge needles
- 5−10 mL lidocaine 1%
- Towel
- Specimen bottles
- Gauze
- Tape
- Sharps bin: the sharps bin should always be taken to the point of care

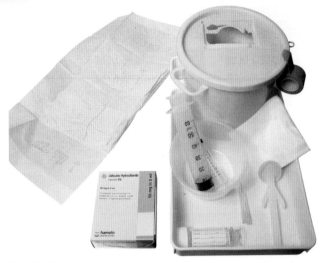

Fig. 5.4 The number of specimen bottles required depends on the investigations you are going to order. It is better to fill too many bottles than not have enough.

Note: Skin-cleansing solutions and method will vary depending on local policy.

EXPLAINING A KNEE JOINT ASPIRATION TO THE PATIENT

1. A knee joint aspiration is a procedure that will allow us to obtain a sample of fluid which has built up in your knee.
2. Local anaesthetic (LA) is injected around the area of skin where the needle is inserted to numb the skin and provide pain relief.
3. The sample is then obtained by inserting a needle through the skin and into the affected knee.
4. We will extract a sample of fluid and send it to the laboratory for testing.
5. The needle is then removed and a dressing is put over the area.
6. It is possible that a sample of fluid cannot be obtained using this method, and this may mean that we need to perform the procedure using ultrasound guidance.

PERFORMING A KNEE JOINT ASPIRATION (LATERAL APPROACH)

PREPARATION

1. Ask the patient to lie on the bed and expose their knee.
2. Place a rolled-up towel under the knee joint so it is slightly flexed.
3. Palpate the margins of the knee joint, including the patella and medial joint line.
4. Locate the intended puncture site, which is the intersection point between the lateral and proximal borders of the patella (Fig. 5.5).
5. Pour antiseptic solution into the universal container.

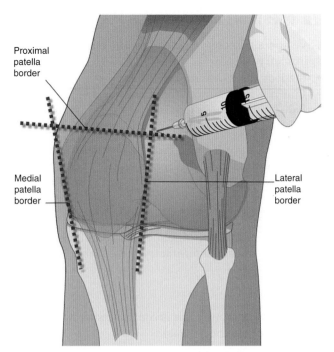

Fig. 5.5 Note the important anatomical landmarks (labelled) when aspirating a knee joint.

6. Wash hands, don sterile apron and gloves.
7. Clean site using gauze soaked in antiseptic solution, from the intended site of puncture outwards. Allow to dry fully.
8. Attach the 21-gauge needle to the 10-mL syringe and draw up 5–10 mL of lidocaine 1% into the knee joint at the intended puncture site. This is done by slowly inserting the needle whilst concurrently aspirating back to ensure you have not hit a blood vessel.

ASPIRATION

1. Attach the second 21-gauge needle to the 30–60 mL syringe.
2. Insert the needle into the soft tissue between the patella and femur at the intended puncture site.
3. Direct the needle at a 45-degree angle towards the midline of the medial side of the joint.
4. Once correctly in place, aspirate the synovial fluid.
5. Once the syringe is filled with synovial fluid, remove the needle and syringe from the knee joint.
6. Apply pressure to the puncture site using gauze and secure with tape.
7. Dispose of needle in the sharps bin.
8. Transfer the fluid into the specimen bottles and label at the bedside.
9. Inform the patient to let a member of staff know if the site is painful, bleeds or if they have any other concerns.
10. Explain that they can remove the dressing after a couple of hours.
11. Remove gloves, and wash hands.
12. Document the procedure in the patient's notes.

DOCUMENTING THE PROCEDURE

Document under the following headings:
- Knee joint aspiration performed
- Indications for the procedure
- Patient consent
- Relevant laboratory investigations; for example, international normalized ratio (INR)/prothrombin time (PT), platelet count
- Procedure technique, sterile preparation, anaesthetic and amount used, amount of fluid obtained, appearance of fluid obtained, estimated blood loss

- Complications
- Subsequent tests ordered, if any, e.g. computed tomography (CT), ultrasound (USS)

Present Your Findings

Mr Jenner is a 62-year-old man who has presented with an acute swollen, tender and erythematous red knee. Knee joint aspiration reveals that there was cloudy, yellow fluid built up in his left knee. White cell count (WCC) was approximately 70,000 cells/mm^3, with 90% neutrophils, and Gram stain was positive. This is in keeping with septic arthritis.

Mark Scheme for Examiner

	0	1	2	3
Introduction and General Advice				
Introduces self, and washes hands				
Confirms patient's identity with three points of identification				
Explains procedure, identifies concerns and obtains consent				
Checks for allergies, needle phobia and clotting				
Preparation				
Obtains equipment and checks expiry dates				
Prepares equipment				
Positions the patient				
Locates site of needle insertion				
Washes hands, dons sterile gloves and apron				
Cleans site				
Prepares LA				
Infiltrates intended puncture site with LA				
Aspiration				
Inserts needle and syringe				
Aspirates synovial fluid				
Disposes of sharp immediately				
Applies dressing over puncture site				
Finishing				
Tells patient to inform staff if site becomes painful or bleeds, and that they can remove dressing after a few hours				
Transfers fluid into specimen bottles, labels at bedside				
Disposes of equipment and cleans tray				
Removes gloves and washes hands				
Documents procedure in the patient notes				
General Points				
Talks to the patient throughout the procedure				
Avoids patient contamination (i.e. NTT)				

0= Not attempted
1= Performed, with room for improvement
2= Adequately performed
3= Performed beyond level expected

❓ QUESTIONS AND ANSWERS FOR CANDIDATE

Name two causes of haemarthrosis.
- Trauma
- Haemophilia and other coagulation disorders
- Anticoagulation therapy

What is the 'Ottawa knee rule'?
- A set of criteria used to determine whether an X-ray is needed for patients with suspected knee fracture

Name three risk factors for gout.
- Diet that is rich in meat and shellfish
- Obesity
- Family history of gout
- Male gender
- Increasing age
- Diuretic use
- High alcohol consumption

What is the microscopic difference between gout and pseudogout?
- Gout is due to the build-up of uric acid crystals, which are needle-shaped and are negatively birefringent.
- Pseudogout is due to the build-up of calcium pyrophosphate crystals, which are rhomboid-shaped and (weakly) positively birefringent.

What are the indications for performing a knee joint aspiration?
- Diagnostic:
  - Septic arthritis
  - Gout
  - Pseudogout
- Therapeutic:
  - Effusion
  - Haemarthrosis
- Additionally, medication (for example, steroids) can be injected into the joint to assist in the treatment of tendonitis or bursitis

Tip Box

Relaxation of the quadriceps makes it easier to insert the needle.

Fact Box

There are several different techniques for performing knee joint aspiration. The commonest technique is the lateral approach, described above. Others include the medial approach, which involves entering the joint under the middle of the patella, or the anterior approach.

STATION 5.4: NASOGASTRIC TUBE INSERTION

SCENARIO

Mrs Tregony is an 84-year-old woman who has been admitted following a stroke. She has been fully assessed, and your consultant has asked you to insert a nasogastric (NG) tube as she has an impaired swallow.

Please perform an NG tube insertion, and describe how you would assess the position of the tube.

OBJECTIVES
- Performing NG tube insertion.
- Checking NG tube positioning.

GENERAL ADVICE
- Ensure that your patient has consented to the procedure and there are no contraindications to NG tube insertion.

EQUIPMENT CHECKLIST

(Remember to check expiry dates on all equipment (Fig. 5.6).)
- Non-sterile gloves
- Single-use apron
- Lubricant gel
- NG tube
- 60-mL syringe
- pH strip
- Sticky tape
- Drainage system
- Cup of water
- Optional: LA spray

EXPLAINING AN NG TUBE INSERTION TO THE PATIENT

1. An NG tube is a plastic, flexible tube that is used to give you food and medication directly into the stomach.
2. It is fed through the nostrils and goes down the back of your throat and into the stomach.

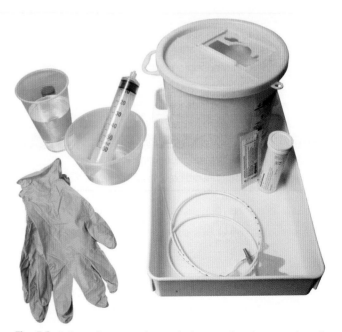
Fig. 5.6 Collect all your equipment before starting the procedure. It may be helpful to have an assistant.

3. This procedure can be carried out on the wards and you will be awake the whole time.
4. It should not be painful, but it may cause some discomfort, especially when the tube gets to the back of your throat.
5. Once it is in, we will verify that the tube has correctly gone into your stomach and only when deemed safe to do so will we give you food and medication through the tube.
6. It is possible the doctor may be unable to insert it into the stomach at the first attempt. If this happens, the doctor will ask your permission before trying again.

INSERTING AN NG TUBE

PREPARATION

1. Introduce yourself to the patient and check consent.
2. Ensure the patient has no allergies to anaesthetic spray (if this is being used).
3. Sit the patient upright with their chin up.
4. Estimate the length of tube required by measuring from the tip of the patient's nose to the xiphisternum, passing via the tragus of the ear (Fig. 5.7).
5. Wash hands, and don sterile gloves and apron.

NG TUBE INSERTION

1. Lubricate the end 5–8 cm of the tube with lubricant gel.
2. Slide the tube along the floor of the nasal cavity initially aiming towards the occiput. There is usually slight resistance as the tube passes into the oesophagus (Fig. 5.8).
3. Ask the patient to swallow repeatedly or offer sips of water to assist with tube insertion.
4. Advance the tube to the predetermined distance and then aspirate stomach fluid using the syringe.
5. Assess the positioning of the tube using pH indicator paper.
6. Tape the tube securely to the patient's nose, and document the length of tube inserted at the nostril entry point.
7. Attach the tube to a drainage system or spigot off as directed.

VERIFYING THE CORRECT POSITION

Method 1 – pH Testing
(Usually a safe method if the tube is only being used for drainage.)
1. Aspirate the contents of the NG tube using a sterile oral syringe.
2. Place a small amount of the aspirated contents on pH indicator paper.
3. Check the pH reading (Fig. 5.9).

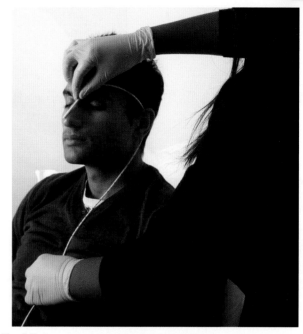

Fig. 5.7 Correctly measure the NG tube before insertion.

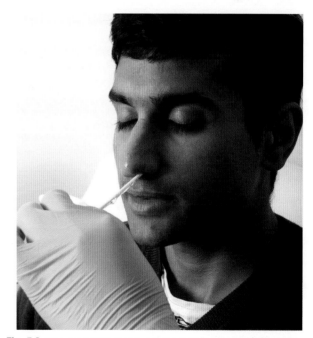

Fig. 5.8 Constantly talk to the patient when inserting an NG tube.

Method 2 – Chest X-ray
- This method is indicated if the pH reading is >5.5 or if there is any doubt with regard to the position of the NG tube.
- A chest X-ray including the upper abdomen is required to locate the tip of the NG tube (which is radiopaque).

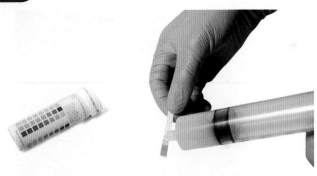

Fig. 5.9 pH testing must be undertaken before an NG tube can be used.

FINISHING

1. Remove the guidewire (if the NG tube has one).
2. Fix the tube in place using tape.
3. Remove gloves, and wash hands.
4. Inform the patient that the procedure is complete, and to speak to a member of staff if they feel any discomfort or have any further questions.
5. Document the procedure in the patient's notes.

DOCUMENTING THE PROCEDURE

Document under the following headings:
- NG tube inserted
- Indications for the procedure
- Patient consent
- Allergy status
- Procedure technique
- Complications.
- Subsequent tests ordered e.g. chest X-ray, litmus strip test for pH

Present Your Findings

Today I inserted an NG tube for Mrs Tregony, who has recently had a stroke and was deemed to have an unsafe swallow. The insertion was relatively easy; however, aspirate was unattainable. Therefore a chest X-ray was requested and it confirmed that the NG tube is definitely in the stomach, so it is safe to use.

Mark Scheme for Examiner

	0	1	2	3
Introduction and General Advice				
Introduces self and washes hands				
Confirms patient's identity with three points of identification				
Explains procedure, identifies concerns and obtains consent				
Checks for allergies				
Preparation				
Obtains equipment and checks expiry dates				
Prepares equipment				
Positions the patient				
Dons single-use apron				
Washes hands and dons sterile gloves				
Estimates NG tube length				
NG Tube Insertion				
Lubricates tube				
Slides tube along nasal cavity to predetermined distance (asking patient to swallow during advancement)				
Verifying Position — pH Testing				
Aspirates contents				
Assesses with pH paper				
Verifying Position — Chest X-Ray				
Orders chest X-ray to identify position				
Finishing				
Removes the guidewire				
Decompresses the stomach				
Disposes of equipment				
Removes gloves and washes hands				
Documents procedure in the patient's notes				
General Points				
Talks to the patient throughout the procedure				

0= Not attempted
1= Performed, with room for improvement
2= Adequately performed
3= Performed beyond level expected

❓ QUESTIONS AND ANSWERS FOR CANDIDATE

What are the common indications for NG tube insertion?
- Feeding (supplementing oral intake or where oral intake is not possible)
- To empty the upper gastrointestinal tract; for example, bowel obstruction

What are the contraindications to NG tube insertion?
- Nasal trauma
- Base-of-skull fracture
- Postoperative upper gastrointestinal surgery patient. If a patient requires an NG tube in this setting, it will be inserted at the time of surgery. If the NG needs to be replaced, for any reason, this should be discussed with the senior surgeons overseeing their care

When should the position of the NG tube be confirmed?
- Immediately after initial placement
- Following significant vomiting or coughing
- If the patient complains of significant pain

How long can a tube stay in situ before needing to be replaced?
- Up to 6 weeks

What method is available to someone who requires long-term enteral feeding?
- Percutaneous endoscopic gastrostomy

 Tip Box

If the patient coughs excessively, the tube could be incorrectly placed. Withdraw the tube and attempt to repeat the insertion.

 Fact Box

There are several substances that can affect the pH of the stomach contents; for example, recent intake of milk, proton pump inhibitors (PPIs) and proton (H_2) receptor antagonists. These should be taken into account when interpreting the pH result.

STATION 5.5: DIAGNOSTIC PLEURAL TAP

SCENARIO

Mrs Haines is a 52-year-old woman who presents with shortness of breath, fatigue and bloating. She admits that she had some weight loss and menstrual irregularities. The respiratory examination demonstrates stony dull percussion on the right side and shifting dullness on abdominal percussion. Subsequent radiological investigations demonstrate a right-sided pleural effusion. Pelvic examination reveals the presence of a mass. Please perform a diagnostic aspiration of the pleural effusion, and then interpret the findings.

OBJECTIVES
- Perform a pleural tap
- Interpret the results

GENERAL ADVICE
- Obtain consent.
- An USS should be performed as part of the assessment for a suspected pleural effusion.
- British Thoracic Society guidelines currently recommend the use of bedside ultrasound guidance for any pleural procedures such as diagnostic pleural taps as it increases the likelihood of success and reduces the risk of adverse events.

EQUIPMENT CHECKLIST

(Remember to check expiry dates on all equipment.)
- Sterile gloves
- Single-use apron
- Three skin-cleansing swabs
- 25-gauge needle
- Three 21-gauge needles
- 10-mL syringe (for LA)
- 50-mL syringe (for pleural aspirate)
- Sterile pack with sterile towels and drape
- 10 mL lidocaine 1%
- Sterile dressing
- Sticky tape
- Sterile specimen bottles (usually three plus a glucose bottle)
- Sharps bin: the sharps bin should always be taken to the point of care

Note: Skin-cleansing solutions and method will vary depending on local policy.

EXPLAINING A PLEURAL TAP TO THE PATIENT

1. A pleural tap is a procedure that allows us to obtain a sample of fluid which has built up in the space between your lungs and ribs. It is usually performed under ultrasound guidance.
2. Local anaesthetic is injected around the area of skin where the needle is inserted to numb the skin and provide some pain relief.

3. The sample is then obtained by inserting a needle through the skin and into the space between your ribs and lungs.
4. We will extract a sample of fluid, and send it to the laboratory for testing.
5. The needle is then removed and a dressing put over the area.
6. We may need to obtain a chest X-ray afterwards (to check for any leakage of air from the lungs).
7. It is possible that a sample of fluid cannot be obtained using this method, and this may mean that we need to perform the procedure using ultrasound guidance.

PERFORMING A PLEURAL TAP

PREPARATION

1. Introduce yourself to the patient and obtain consent.
2. Assemble the equipment.
3. Expose the patient from head to waist.
4. Position the patient sitting upright on the bed, with pillows on a nearby table to support their arms (Fig. 5.10).
5. Listen to the chest to determine the site and size of the pleural effusion.
6. Percuss the upper border of the effusion and choose a site one or two interspaces below that upper border, in the mid-clavicular line.
7. Open the sterile pack and arrange all equipment into the sterilised field using an aseptic technique.

ASEPTIC TECHNIQUE

1. Wash hands, and don sterile gloves and apron.
2. Attach the 21-gauge needle to the 10-mL syringe and draw up 5–10 mL of lidocaine 1%. Attach the 25-gauge needle and keep one 21-gauge needle ready for deeper infiltration.
3. Attach the third 21-gauge needle to a 50-mL syringe ready for pleural aspiration.
4. Place all needles and syringe sets in the sterile field.
5. Put the drape on the patient with the open window over the target area.
6. Mark the site and clean the area with skin-cleansing swabs in a spiral pattern 3 times.
7. Inject LA: use the 25-gauge needle to anaesthetise the skin superficially.
8. Swap the 25-gauge with the 21-gauge needle and anaesthetise down to the pleura. Once anaesthetised, note needle depth, and then withdraw the needle and syringe, disposing into sharps bin. Then insert the 21-gauge needle (attached to the 50-mL syringe), **aspirating whilst advancing** the needle.
9. Draw up 10–20 mL of pleural fluid (Fig. 5.11).

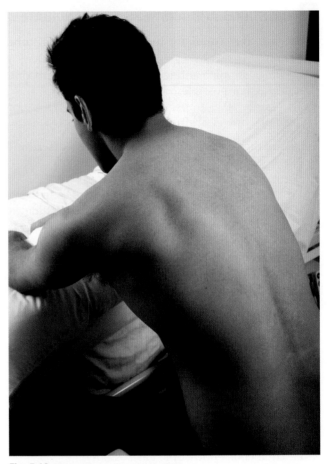

Fig. 5.10 Correctly position the patient.

10. Withdraw the needle and place into the sterilised field.
11. Apply pressure with a sterile dressing and then tape the dressing into place.
12. Transfer the aspirate into a sterile universal container and send to the laboratory for:
    - Chemistry: protein, glucose, pH, lactate dehydrogenase (LDH), amylase
    - Bacteriology: microscopy, culture and sensitivity (MC&S)
13. If indicated, consider sending the sample for:
    - Acid-fast staining (if tuberculosis (TB) is suspected)
    - Immunology (rheumatoid factor, antinuclear antibodies, complement)
    - Cytology

VENOUS BLOOD SAMPLE

A venous blood sample can be taken for serum protein and LDH. This is to compare the protein and LDH in the pleural space with that in the blood (using Light's criteria), and to determine whether the pleural aspirate

• Subsequent tests ordered, if any, e.g. chest X-ray, CT, USS

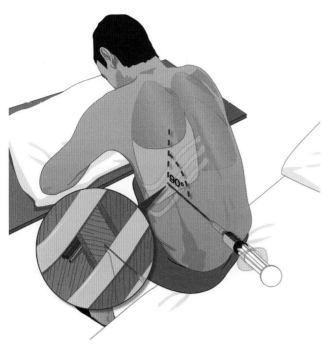

Fig. 5.11 Correct positioning for pleural aspiration. The needle should be inserted perpendicular to the skin (drape not shown).

is exudative or transudative. A capillary glucose is also helpful for this reason.

DOCUMENTING THE PROCEDURE

Document under the following headings:
• Pleural tap performed
• Indications for the procedure
• Patient consent
• Relevant laboratory investigations; for example, INR/PT, platelet count
• Procedure technique, sterile preparation, anaesthetic and amount used, amount of fluid obtained, appearance of fluid obtained, estimated blood loss
• Complications

Risks of Performing a Pleural Tap

Common (>5%)	Uncommon (1%–5%)	Rare (<1%)
• Pneumothorax • Infection (wound or chest) • Fainting (vasovagal)	• Pain • Shortness of breath	• Haemothorax • Damage to nearby structures (i.e. liver, spleen, colon) • Death

Interpreting a Pleural Aspirate
(Without Comparison to Blood Sample Values)

Transudate (protein <30 g/L)	Exudative (protein >30 g/L)
Caused by the 'failures' and low-protein states: • Liver failure/cirrhosis • Heart failure • Nephrotic syndrome • Hypothyroidism • Fluid overload • Meigs syndrome	• Pneumonia • TB • Malignancy • PE

Present Your Findings

Mrs Haines presented with a right-sided pleural effusion and a diagnostic pleural tap was performed which revealed a pleural protein level of 45 g/L, confirming that it is an exudate. Other results included pleural LDH > 1000 IU/L and a low pleural fluid level as well as a low pH. These results are consistent with a malignancy, which is likely the cause of the pleural effusion.

Mark Scheme for Examiner

	0	1	2	3
Introduction and General Advice				
Introduces self, and washes hands				
Confirms patient's identity with three points of identification				
Explains procedure, identifies concerns and obtains consent				
Checks chest X-ray and USS				
Positions and exposes patient				
Identifies spot marked for pleural tap				
Percusses and auscultates to check location of effusion				

Continued

Mark Scheme for Examiner—cont'd

	0	1	2	3
Preparation				
Obtains equipment and checks expiry dates				
Prepares equipment				
Washes hands, dons sterile gloves and apron				
Places drape over the patient				
Cleans site in a spiral pattern 3 times				
Performing the Pleural Tap				
Injects LA using the 'withdraw and infiltrate' method				
Withdraws needle and syringe				
Inserts another needle and withdraws up to 50 mL of aspirate				
Applies pressure to insertion site and places dressing				
Finishing				
Labels specimen bottles at the bedside				
Disposes of all sharps immediately				
Disposes of equipment and cleans tray				
Removes gloves, and washes hands				
Documents procedure in the patient notes				
General Points				
Talks to the patient throughout the procedure				
Avoids patient contamination (i.e. NTT)				

0= Not attempted
1= Performed, with room for improvement
2= Adequately performed
3= Performed beyond level expected

❓ QUESTIONS AND ANSWERS FOR CANDIDATE

What is the difference between pleural effusion and pulmonary oedema?

- A pleural effusion is fluid build-up in the space in between the parietal and visceral pleura of the lung. Pulmonary oedema is fluid leakage into the lung interstitium and alveoli.

What is the difference between transudative and exudative pleural effusions?

- Transudates occur with a structurally normal pleura, but raised oncotic and hydrostatic pressure results in fluid leak.
- Exudates occur with a damaged pleura, resulting in loss of tissue fluid and protein.

What are some common causes of an exudative pleural effusion?

- Malignancy
- Pulmonary embolism
- Pneumonia
- TB

What are Light's criteria?

- Light's criteria are used to determine if the patient's type of pleural effusion is transudative or exudative, by comparing pleural fluid with blood.

 Tip Box

Pleural taps are usually performed under ultrasound guidance. It is advisable to stay at or above the eighth intercostal space (T8) to avoid the liver and the spleen and to stay below the tip of the scapula by at least 5 cm.

 Fact Box

All needles should be inserted perpendicular to the skin directly above the upper edge of the corresponding rib into the pleural space occupied by the pleural fluid. This minimises the risk of the needle damaging the neurovascular bundle, which runs along the underside of the rib.

STATION 5.6: CHEST DRAIN

SCENARIO

Mr Lodger is a 58-year-old man who has been in the intensive therapy unit (ITU) following admission to hospital for severe community-acquired pneumonia. The respiratory examination demonstrates decreased air entry and stony dull percussion on the left side. A significant left-sided pleural effusion is confirmed on USS, and the decision is made to drain this collection via pleurocentesis. Please insert a chest drain.

OBJECTIVES

- Insert a thoracic chest drain
- Connect the drain correctly to the chest drain bottle
- Understand the principles of how to assess a correctly functioning chest drain

GENERAL ADVICE

- Obtain consent.
- Inspect the chest X-ray and USS to detect the size and site of the pleural effusion.
- Remember to adjust the position of the chest drain with regard to drainage of either pleural fluid or pneumothorax.
- Always keep sight of the guidewire when using the Seldinger technique. One hand should always ensure that an adequate length of wire is available outside the patient.
- Do not force the dilators or chest drain tube as this may lead to kinking of the guidewire and create false passages.
- Check the patient's blood results before doing the procedure, particularly the platelet count and clotting function. Bloods for albumin, protein, LDH and glucose are helpful in interpreting pleural fluid tests.
- If the patient feels faint during the procedure, stop and withdraw the needle immediately and lay the patient down.
- We have shown the procedure for drain insertion using a typical Seldinger kit, but the choice of tube or method should always be considered. For example, wide-bore tubes should always be used in preference to Seldinger tubes in trauma where it is felt the latter would provide inadequate drainage of blood.

EQUIPMENT CHECKLIST

(Remember to check expiry dates on all equipment.)
- An assistant
- Water-tight universal drain container with sterile tubing and connector
- Sterile water
- Chest drainage catheter equipment:
  - Introducer needle
  - Guidewire
  - Dilators
  - Chest drain
  - Four-way tap
  - Male connector
- Single-use apron
- Sterile gloves
- Skin-cleansing swabs and spray
- Suture pack and suture
- Scalpel
- 10-mL syringe, 25-gauge needle and two 21-gauge needles (for LA)
- 10 mL lidocaine 1%
- Sterile pack with sterile towels and drape
- Sharps bin: the sharps bin should always be taken to the point of care
- Sterile trolley
- Sterile dressing

Note: Skin-cleansing solutions and method will vary depending on local policy.

EXPLAINING A CHEST DRAIN TO THE PATIENT

1. A chest drain is a plastic tube which allows us to drain fluid or air from the space which has built up between your lungs and ribs.
2. Local anaesthetic is injected around the area of skin where the needle is inserted to numb the skin and provide some pain relief.
3. A guidewire is inserted through a needle in the skin into the space between your ribs and lungs.
4. The entry site is then widened, and a plastic tube is inserted through the guidewire so that it is in the correct place.
5. The other side of the plastic tube is connected to a plastic container with water inside that will allow any fluid or air to be drained.
6. The plastic tube is secured with stitches and a dressing is put over the insertion area.
7. We will need to obtain chest X-rays afterwards to check that the drain is in the right position.

INSERTING A CHEST DRAIN

PREPARATION

1. Introduce yourself to the patient and obtain written consent.
2. Arrange all the equipment on a sterile trolley ready to be opened.
3. Assemble the underwater seal by filling the universal chest drain container with an adequate amount of sterile water. Position the container near your assistant and the sterile tubing on the sterile trolley.
4. Expose the patient from head to waist and position the patient sitting slightly rotated upright on the bed, with pillows cascaded below the shoulder and upper back.
5. Spray the patient adequately with chlorhexidine spray down the mid-axillary line, plus front and back around the safe triangle. Leave to air dry (Fig. 5.12).

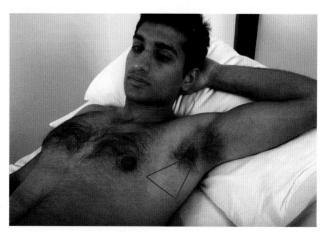

Fig. 5.12 The safe triangle for insertion.

INSERTION

1. Scrub up aseptically, and put on sterile apron and gloves.
2. Open the sterile pack and arrange all equipment into the sterile field using an aseptic technique.
3. Attach the chest drain to the four-way tap and male connector, and turn the rotator on the tap to prevent any air entering the drain (Fig. 5.13).
4. Attach the 21-gauge needle to the 10-mL syringe and draw up 5—10 mL of lidocaine 1%.
5. Clean the skin with chlorhexidine swabs in a spiral pattern 3 times.
6. Drape the patient in a 'box' fashion with a clear view of the 'safety triangle' (Fig. 5.14).
7. Determine the fourth or fifth intercostal space in the 'safe triangle'.
8. Infiltrate the proposed area for drain insertion with LA. Use the 25-gauge needle to anaesthetise the skin superficially. Swap the 25-gauge with the second 21-gauge needle and anaesthetise down to the pleura, using the 'infiltrate and aspirate' method. Keep note of the depth of the needle when pleural fluid is aspirated.

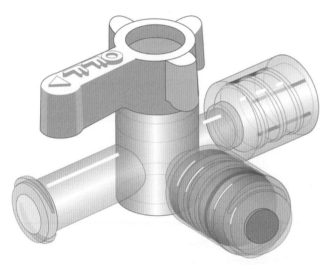

Fig. 5.13 Correct position of the tap to prevent air entering the chest.

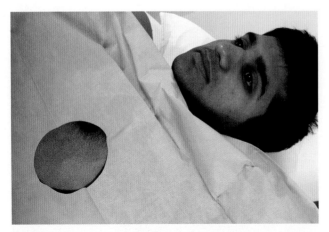

Fig. 5.14 Draping the patient with adequate clearance.

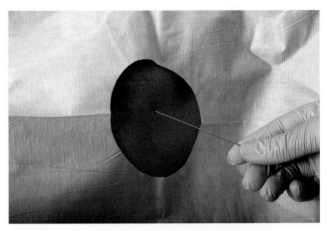

Fig. 5.15 Correct positioning for introducer needle.

9. Withdraw the needle and dispose of it in the sharps bin.
10. Swap the 21-gauge needle with the introducer needle (now attached to the syringe), and redetermine the rib just below the intercostal space you intend to enter.
11. Insert the introducer needle, aiming just above the upper border of the rib just palpated (Fig. 5.15).
12. Stop advancing when pleural fluid or air is aspirated. This should be a similar depth to that noted previously.
13. If no pleural fluid or free air is aspirated, do not continue with the chest tube without further imaging guidance.
14. Stabilise the introducer needle against the skin with your non-dominant hand to ensure that it remains immobile from this position.

Insertion of the Chest Drain Seldinger

1. Pick up the guidewire with your dominant hand, and with your thumb pull back on the guidewire so the curved tip is now barely visible past the plastic cover. This is to straighten the tip of the guidewire.
2. Detach the syringe from the introducer. Insert the plastic top of the guidewire into the opening of the introducer needle, and feed the guidewire into the pleural space with your thumb.
3. Remove the plastic sheath from the guidewire when approximately 10 cm remains and grab the guidewire with your non-dominant hand (Fig. 5.16).
4. Remove the introducer needle from the skin by pulling it out over the guidewire, and place it on the sterile tray with your dominant hand.
5. Withdraw and reinsert the guidewire slightly to ensure that it moves freely.
6. Make a small horizontal and vertical incision at the insertion point of the guidewire with the tip of the scalpel.
7. Set the maximum penetration depth of the dilators using the depth previously noted during insertion of the introducer needle.

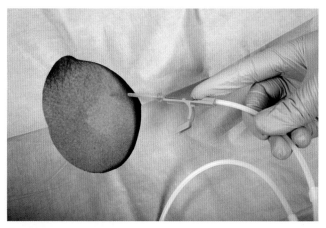

Fig. 5.16 Removing the plastic sheath from the guidewire.

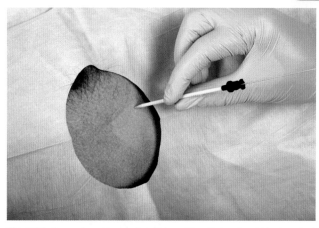

Fig. 5.17 Correct positioning for dilators. The dilator should be inserted perpendicular to the skin following the same tract as the needle and guidewire previously.

8. Securing the guidewire's tip gently with your non-dominant hand, thread the first dilator through the guidewire until its set depth (Fig. 5.17).
9. Repeat this process with the other dilators of increasing diameter.
10. Remove the last dilator, and secure the guidewire's tip gently with your non-dominant hand.

11. Ensure that the tap at the end of the chest drain is closed to the outside environment to prevent air from entering the pleural cavity.
12. Insert the chest drain over the guidewire perpendicular to the skin.

Securing the chest drain

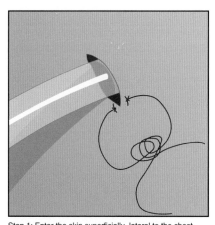

Step 1: Enter the skin superficially, lateral to the chest tube on one side at its lower border with the suture, and exit the skin just above the entrance site at the upper border of the chest tube on the same side

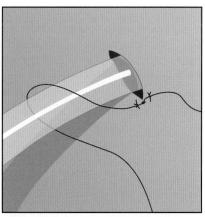

Step 2: Pull the suture through the wound so there is an equal amount of string on both sides and tie a reef knot. Cut the needle from the suture and lay it on the sterile table for disposal later

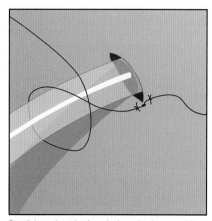

Step 3: Loop the string from the lower border around the chest drain several times

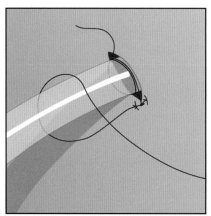

Step 4: Loop the string from the upper border around the chest drain several times. The two ends should remain on opposite sides afterwards

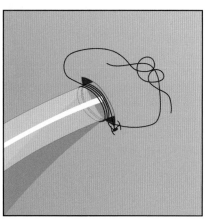

Step 5: Tie another reef knot

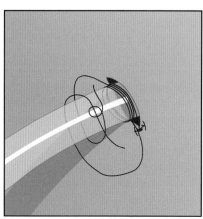

Step 6: Wrap the remaining strings around the tube and tie another reef knot

Tying a reef knot

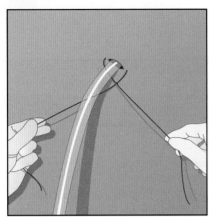

Step 1: Hold the suture ends (RED in left hand, BLUE in right hand), ensuring the suture is wrapped around the back of the chest drain tubing

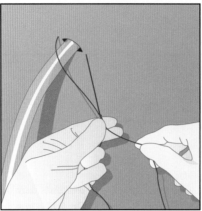

Step 2: Put the blue suture over the top of the red suture and hold the point where they meet with your left hand

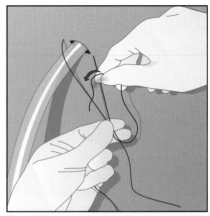

Step 3: With your right hand take the red suture end. Lift it up in the air, and then bring it down from above through the triangle formed by the sutures being crossed over

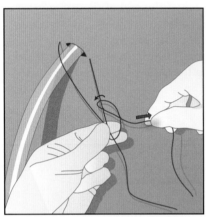

Step 4: After going down vertically down through the triangle, bring the red suture end out from the underside of the triangle, to the right

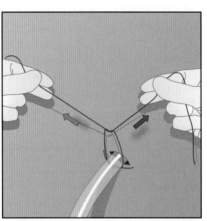

Step 5: Pull two suture ends. The sutures should lie flat against the skin

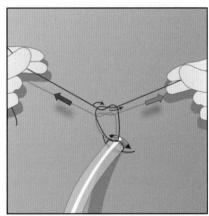

Step 6: Repeat the steps above to form a flat sitting

FINISHING

1. Apply two dressings in a 'duck bill' fashion above and below the chest drain.
2. Connect the male end of the chest drain to the sterile tubing whilst ensuring that the chest drain does not dislodge from the patient.
3. Ask your assistant to open the watertight universal drain container and present it to you.
4. Place the rigid part of the sterile tubing through the opening. Ensure you remain sterile throughout this part of the procedure and that the chest drain does not dislodge from the patient (Fig. 5.18).
5. Ensure that the rigid sterile tubing is well immersed in the sterile water but not obstructed by the bottom of the container.
6. Check that the chest tube is draining the pleural effusion or bubbling is seen underwater in the sterile container.
7. Remove the sterile drapes and dispose of any sharps.
8. Order a post-procedure chest X-ray to review the position of the chest drain.

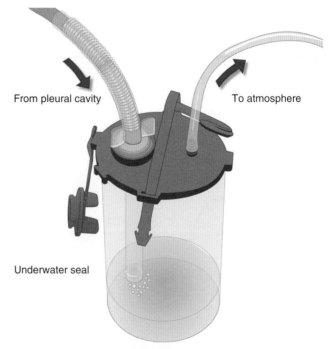

From pleural cavity

To atmosphere

Underwater seal

Fig. 5.18 Inserting the chest drain tubing into the watertight drain container held by the assistant.

DOCUMENTING THE PROCEDURE

Document under the following headings:
- Chest drain inserted
- Indications for the procedure
- Patient consent
- Relevant laboratory investigations (e.g. clotting, platelet count)
- Procedure technique, sterile preparation, anaesthetic use, amount of fluid obtained, appearance of fluid obtained, estimated blood loss
- Complications
- Subsequent tests ordered, if any (e.g. chest X-ray, CT, USS)

Indications for Performing a Chest Drain

Pneumothorax	Others
• In any ventilated patient • Tension pneumothorax after initial needle relief • Persistent or recurrent pneumothorax after simple aspiration • Large, secondary spon-taneous pneumothorax in patients aged >50	• Malignant pleural effusion • Empyema and complicated parapneumonic pleural effusion • Traumatic haemopneumothorax • Postoperative — after thoracotomy, oesophagectomy of cardiac surgery (usually performed at the time of surgery)

Mark Scheme for Examiner

	0	1	2	3
Introduction and General Advice				
Introduces self, and washes hands				
Confirms patient's identity with three points of identification				
Explains procedure, identifies concerns and obtains consent				
Checks chest X-ray and USS, clotting and platelet count				
Positions and exposes patient				
Describes safe triangle and sprays with chlorhexidine				
Preparation				
Obtains equipment and checks expiry dates				
Prepares equipment				
Washes hands, dons sterile gloves and apron				
Sets up equipment in a logical fashion within hand reach				
Places drape over the patient				
Cleans site in a spiral pattern 3 times				
Inserting the Chest Drain				
Identifies fourth/fifth intercostal space in the safe triangle				
Injects LA using the 'withdraw and infiltrate' method				
Inserts introducer needle				
Withdraws straw-coloured aspirate or free air during deep infiltration				
Secures introducer needle and removes syringe				
Inserts the guidewire and keeps it secure. Removes introducer				
Appropriately dilates and blunt dissects the insertion point				
Rechecks that tap at the end of the chest drain is closed to air				
Inserts chest drain over guidewire				
Closes the wound and sutures the chest drain securely				
Attaches the chest drain to the drain container and checks for bubbling and aspiration of pleural fluid				
Finishing				
Disposes of all sharps immediately				
Disposes of equipment				
Removes drapes and gloves, and washes hands				
Documents procedure in the patient notes				
Orders postprocedure chest X-ray				

Continued

Mark Scheme for Examiner—cont'd

	0	1	2	3
General Points				
Talks to the patient throughout the procedure				
Avoids patient contamination (i.e. NTT)				

0= Not attempted
1= Performed, with room for improvement
2= Adequately performed
3= Performed beyond level expected

❓ QUESTIONS AND ANSWERS FOR CANDIDATE

Are abnormal blood clotting or platelet counts contraindications for insertion of a chest drain?

• There is currently no evidence that demonstrates bleeding complications of chest drain insertions due to abnormal clotting or platelet counts. However, these should be corrected where possible as good practice.

Why should the chest drain tube be attached to an underwater seal?

• The underwater seal allows draining of the pleural spaces and prevents backflow of air or fluid into the pleural cavity.

Why is the 'safe triangle' recommended for chest drain insertion?

• It minimises the risk of injury to internal organs and vascular structures, e.g. the internal mammary artery.

What is the maximum volume of fluid that should be drained out in one sitting?

• No more than 1–1.5 L, due to a theoretical risk of re-expansion pulmonary oedema

What is a chylothorax?

• Collection of lymph fluid in the pleural space

💡 Tip Box

Adequate draping helps to eliminate the passage of microorganisms between sterile and non-sterile surfaces. Therefore, any unsterile surfaces (e.g. tubes, patient clothing) should be covered by the drape and not be visible or accessible during the remainder of the aseptic procedure.

🦏 Fact Box

The 'safe triangle' is bordered by the:
• Lateral border of the pectoralis major
• Anterior border of the latissimus dorsi
• Superiorly, by the apex below the axilla
• Inferiorly, by the line at the horizontal level of the nipple

STATION 5.7: DIAGNOSTIC ASCITIC TAP

SCENARIO

Mr Brody is a 48-year-old man who presents to his primary care physician with difficulty breathing, abdominal distension and cachexia. A long-standing history of alcohol abuse is discovered along with shifting dullness and a fluid thrill. Subsequent investigations demonstrate a cirrhotic liver and gross abdominal ascites. Please perform a diagnostic aspiration of the ascites and interpret your findings.

OBJECTIVES

• Perform a diagnostic ascitic tap
• Interpret the results

GENERAL ADVICE

• Obtain consent.
• Ultrasound guidance is recommended to mark the ideal location for an ascitic tap. This ensures that the procedure can be performed as successfully and safely as possible. The following information may also be helpful and ideally should be requested from the sonographer before the procedure:
  • Distance from skin to fluid (in cm)
  • Distance from skin to the midpoint of the collection
• An abdominal USS will also provide information about the likely underlying aetiology, including the presence of lymphadenopathy, splenomegaly and portal hypertension.
• Ensure that the patient has passed urine before the procedure.
• Ensure that you have undertaken a full history and examination on the patient, making note of any clotting disorders. Before starting the procedure make sure you have checked the results of the patient's recent clotting screen and platelet count. At the time of ascitic tap, perform venepuncture. Check serum protein, albumin, urea and electrolyte (U&Es), glucose, LDH (to determine if transudate or exudate) plus any additional tests that may be considered.

EQUIPMENT CHECKLIST

(Remember to check expiry dates on all equipment.)
• Sterile gloves
• Single-use apron
• Three skin-cleansing swabs
• 21-gauge needle
• 50-mL syringe (for ascitic aspirate)

- Sterile pack with sterile towels and drape
- Sterile universal container
- Sterile gauze
- Sterile dressing
- Sharps bin: the sharps bin should always be taken to the point of care

Note: Skin-cleansing solutions and method will vary depending on local policy.

EXPLAINING A DIAGNOSTIC ASCITIC TAP TO THE PATIENT

1. An ascitic tap is a procedure that allows us to obtain a sample of fluid present inside your tummy.
2. You may have to have an ultrasound scan of your abdomen before the procedure, and the radiologist will mark the spot where we take the sample from.
3. The sample is then obtained by inserting a needle through the skin, into the space between your abdominal organs where the fluid has leaked.
4. The fluid obtained is then sent to the laboratory for testing.
5. The needle is then removed and a dressing put over that area.
6. Although unlikely, it may not be possible to obtain a sample of fluid.

PERFORMING AN ASCITIC TAP

PREPARATION

1. Introduce yourself to the patient and obtain written consent.
2. Gather your equipment.
3. Expose the patient's abdomen.
4. Position the patient supine on the bed, with their hands under their head.
5. Percuss the area around the spot marked for the ascitic tap, ensuring that the marked spot corresponds with dullness.
6. Open the sterile pack, and arrange all equipment into the sterile field using an aseptic technique.

ASEPTIC TECHNIQUE

1. Wash hands, and don sterile gloves and single-use apron.
2. Apply sterile drapes. Clean the insertion area in a spiral pattern 3 times, using chlorhexidine swabs (Fig. 5.19).
3. Place all equipment in the sterile field.
4. Attach the 21-gauge needle to a 50-mL syringe for ascitic aspiration.
5. Advance the 21-gauge needle and 50 mL into the abdomen until ascitic fluid is aspirated and draw up to 500 mL of ascitic fluid (Fig. 5.20).
6. Withdraw the needle and place it in the sterile field.
7. Apply pressure with sterile gauze and then cover with a sterile dressing if required.

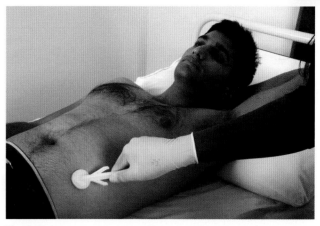

Fig. 5.19 This is a sterile procedure so careful preparation is required.

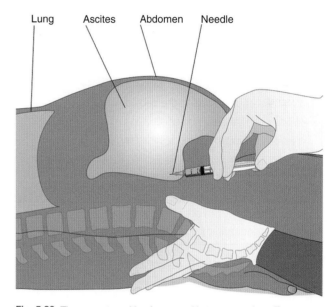

Fig. 5.20 The correct position for an ascitic tap procedure. Ensure you have percussed the abdomen before the procedure.

8. Transfer aspirate into a sterile universal container and send it to the laboratory for:
   - Albumin, protein, LDH, glucose
   - Absolute WCC
9. If indicated, consider sending the sample for:
   - Cytology (if underlying malignancy is suspected)
   - Acid-fast staining (for TB)

DOCUMENT THE PROCEDURE

Document under the following headings:
- Ascitic tap performed
- Indications for the procedure
- Patient consent
- Relevant laboratory investigations; for example, INR/PT, platelet count
- Procedure technique, sterile preparation, anaesthetic and amount used, amount of fluid obtained, appearance of fluid obtained, estimated blood loss

Mark Scheme for Examiner

	0	1	2	3
Introduction and General Advice				
Introduces self, and washes hands				
Confirms patient's identity with three points of identification				
Explains procedure, identifies concerns and obtains consent				
Positions and exposes patient				
Checks USS and clotting				
Identifies spot marked ascitic tap, percusses to check				
Preparation				
Obtains equipment and checks expiry dates				
Prepares equipment				
Washes hands, dons sterile gloves and apron				
Places drape over the patient				
Cleans site in a spiral pattern 3 times				
Performing the Ascitic Tap				
Inserts needle and withdraws up to 50 mL of aspirate				
Applies pressure to insertion site and places dressing				
Finishing				
Labels specimen bottles at the bedside				
Disposes of all sharps immediately				
Disposes of equipment and cleans tray				
Removes gloves, and washes hands				
Documents procedure in the patient notes				
General Points				
Talks to the patient throughout the procedure				
Avoids patient contamination (i.e. NTT)				

0= Not attempted
1= Performed, with room for improvement
2= Adequately performed
3= Performed beyond level expected

- Complications
- Subsequent tests ordered

 Present Your Findings

Mr Brody is a 48-year-old man who has liver cirrhosis and abdominal ascites. A diagnostic abdominal tap was performed which revealed straw-coloured fluid with normal ascitic fluid biochemistry and microscopy. Serum ascites albumin gradient (SAAG) was high, suggesting that it is transudative; therefore, the likely cause of the ascites was liver cirrhosis.

 QUESTIONS AND ANSWERS FOR CANDIDATE

What should you always suspect if a patient becomes unwell after an ascitic tap?
- Spontaneous bacterial peritonitis

What are the different grades of ascites?
- Grade 1 = Only detectable by USS
- Grade 2 = Detected by moderate abdominal distension
- Grade 2 = Detected by marked abdominal distension

How is SAAG calculated?
- SAAG = (albumin concentration of serum) − (albumin concentration of ascitic fluid).

What ascitic WCC is diagnostic of spontaneous bacterial peritonitis?
- WCC $>500/mm^3$
- Or if ascitic neutrophil $\geq250/mm^3$

Tip Box

If USS guidance is not available, the insertion site for an ascitic tap is approximately 15 cm laterally to the umbilicus, usually in either the right or left lower abdominal quadrant. It is also possible to insert 2 cm below the umbilicus in the midline, through the linea alba. Avoid areas of prominent superficial veins (caput medusae), scars and palpable masses.

STATION 5.8: THERAPEUTIC PARACENTESIS

SCENARIO

Mrs Walker is a 64-year-old alcoholic woman with large ascites refractory to diuretic therapy. She is complaining of increasing abdominal pain and shortness of breath. Perform a therapeutic ascitic drain to alleviate her symptoms.

OBJECTIVE

- Perform a therapeutic ascitic drain

GENERAL ADVICE

- Obtain consent.
- Ultrasound guidance is recommended to mark the ideal location for an ascitic tap. This ensures that the procedure can be performed as successfully and safely as possible. The following information may also be helpful and ideally should be requested from the sonographer before the procedure:
  - Distance from skin to fluid (in cm)
  - Distance from skin to the midpoint of the collection
- Ensure that the patient has passed urine before the procedure.
- Ensure that the patient has adequate intravenous (IV) access to give albumin if needed.
- Ensure that you have undertaken a full history and examination on the patient, making note of any clotting disorders. Before starting the procedure make sure you have checked the results of the patient's recent clotting screen and platelet count.

EQUIPMENT CHECKLIST

(Remember to check expiry dates on all equipment (Fig. 5.21).)
- Sterile gloves
- Single-use apron
- Sterile drape
- Three skin-cleansing swabs
- 25-gauge needle
- Two 21-gauge needles
- 10-mL syringe (for LA)
- 10 mL lidocaine 1%
- Bonanno catheter and trocar (introducer)

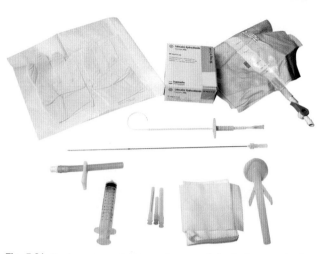

Fig. 5.21 Equipment required to perform an abdominal paracentesis.

- Scalpel (optional)
- Three IV cannula dressings to fix ascitic drain to skin
- 2-L catheter bag and connector tube

EXPLAINING AN ABDOMINAL PARACENTESIS TO THE PATIENT

1. An ascitic drain is a plastic tube that we place through the skin of your belly to allow us to drain away the excess fluid that has accumulated inside.
2. You may have to have an ultrasound scan of your abdomen before the procedure, and the radiologist will mark the spot where we take the sample from.
3. An intravenous line will be placed into your arm, and some blood will also be taken before the procedure.
4. Local anaesthetic is injected around the area of skin where the needle is inserted to numb the skin and provide some pain relief.
5. You may need some fluid via a drip depending on the amount of fluid drained.
6. The drain will be removed after 6 h.

PERFORMING AN ABDOMINAL PARACENTESIS

PREPARATION

1. Introduce yourself to the patient and obtain consent.
2. Cannulate the patient.
3. Gather your equipment and a clean trolley.
4. Expose the patient's abdomen, and ask the patient to keep their hands under their head.
5. Position the patient supine on the bed.
6. Percuss the abdomen and identify the presence of ascites as suggested by shifting dullness. If you are not confident that there is a significant volume of ascites, do not proceed until a point has been marked with ultrasound assistance.

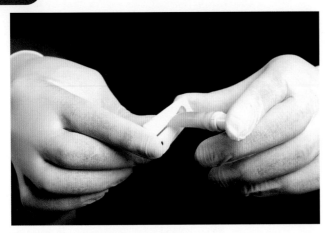

Fig. 5.22 Clamping the connector tube.

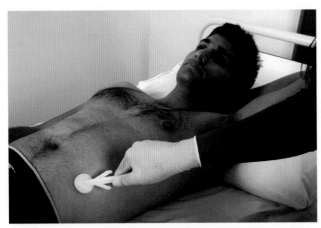

Fig. 5.23 Ensure the abdomen is sterilised for this procedure.

7. Open the sterile pack, and arrange all equipment into the sterile field using an aseptic technique.
8. Clamp the connector tube (Fig. 5.22).

ASEPTIC TECHNIQUE

1. Wash hands and don sterile gloves and apron.
2. Apply sterile drapes.
3. Attach the 21-gauge needle to the 10-mL syringe and draw up 5–10 mL of lidocaine 1%.
4. Mark the site and clean the area with skin-cleansing swabs in a spiral pattern 3 times (Fig. 5.23).
5. Inject LA: use the 25-gauge needle to anaesthetise the skin superficially.
6. Swap the 25-gauge needle with a 21-gauge needle and alternatately aspirate whilst infiltrating LA down towards the peritoneum.
7. Withdraw the LA needle when straw-coloured fluid is easily aspirated, and note the depth of the needle.
8. Prepare the Bonanno catheter by sliding the outer plastic sheath over the catheter to straighten the curved tip (Fig. 5.24).

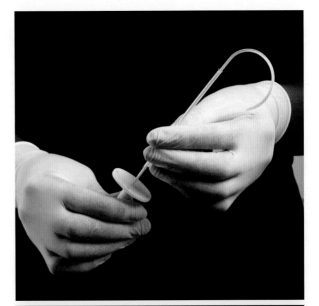

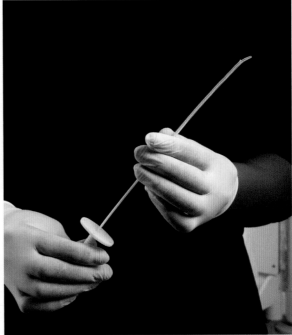

Fig. 5.24 First, straighten the tip by slowly sliding the plastic sheath upwards.

9. Insert the metal trocar inside the catheter and secure it to the catheter base (Fig. 5.25).
10. Completely remove the outer plastic sheath.
11. Carefully push the catheter into the anaesthetised area, keeping full control of the needle at the point of contact at the skin (Fig. 5.26).
12. If excessive force is required to puncture the skin, use the scalpel to make a small incision in the skin to allow the catheter to pass more freely.
13. Continue to advance the catheter into the peritoneal cavity until ascitic fluid can be seen draining back along the needle.

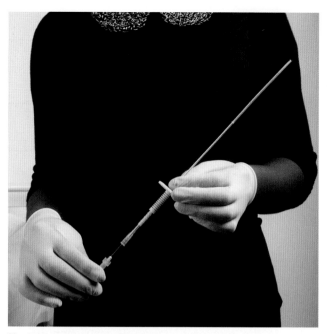

Fig. 5.25 Insert the metal trocar.

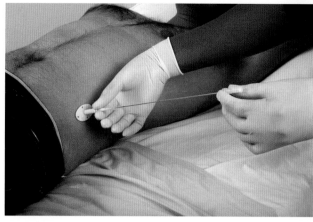

Fig. 5.27 After advancing the catheter, gently remove the trocar.

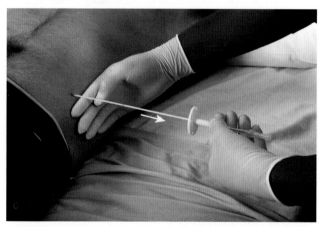

Fig. 5.26 Ensure you have full control over the catheter when you are inserting it.

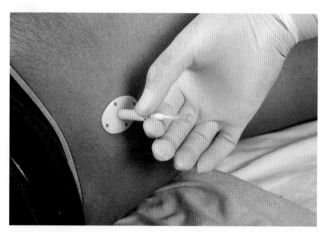

Fig. 5.28 Once the trocar is removed, the plastic tube remains in situ.

14. Advance the needle a further centimetre to ensure the tip of the plastic catheter is within the peritoneal cavity.
15. Unscrew the trocar from the catheter, and advance the catheter over the trocar without moving the trocar any further.
16. Once the catheter is fully inserted, remove the metal trocar (Fig. 5.27). The plastic tube remains in situ (Fig 5.28).
17. Attach the clamped rubber connector tube to the catheter (Fig. 5.29).
18. Connect the catheter bag and place it below the patient (Fig. 5.30).
19. Secure the catheter to the skin using the IV cannula dressings.
20. Unclamp the connector tube and ensure ascites is draining well, and note the colour of the fluid being drained.

DOCUMENTING THE PROCEDURE

Document under the following headings:
* Ascitic drain inserted
* Indications for the procedure
* Patient consent
* Relevant laboratory investigations (e.g. clotting, platelet count)

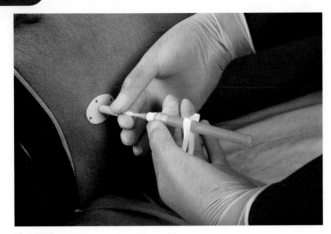

Fig. 5.29 Attach the connecting tubing.

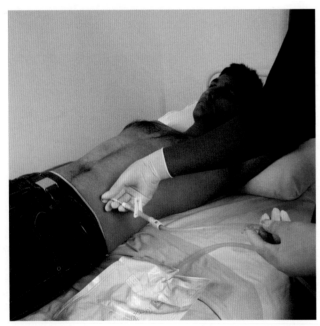

Fig. 5.30 Connect the catheter bag.

- Procedure technique, sterile preparation, anaesthetic and amount used, appearance of fluid obtained
- Complications of an ascitic drain (Table 5.2)
- Time the drain should be removed (usually 6–12 h after insertion)
- Prescribe 100 mL of 20% human albumin solution for every 2–3 L of ascitic fluid drained (depending on local guidelines)

Table 5.2	Complications of an Ascitic Drain	
COMMON (>1%)	**RARE (<0.1%)**
Failure to collect fluid	Haemoperitoneum
Persistent leak from the puncture site	Bowel perforation
Wound infection	Death (due to bleeding or infection)
Abdominal wall haematoma	

❓ QUESTIONS AND ANSWERS FOR CANDIDATE

What is refractory ascites?
- Ascites that fail to respond to intense diuretic therapy
- Ascites that occur in a patient in whom intense diuretic therapy is not tolerated

What is the role of dietary salt restriction in the management of ascites?
- Avoids sodium retention and water overload, which would increase the circulating volume and therefore contribute to portal hypertension

What does TIPS stand for, and what is it?
- TIPS stands for transjugular intrahepatic porto-system shunt.
- It is a connection that is made between two veins within the liver.

Name three indications for a TIPS procedure.
- Secondary prevention of oesophageal variceal bleeding
- Treatment of refractory ascites.
- Portal hypertension gastropathy
- Recurrent acute variceal bleeding
- Budd–Chiari syndrome

What are the risks and benefits of TIPS?

Benefits	Risks
Minimally invasive	Infection
Short recovery time	Bleeding
Little effect on future liver transplantation, if that is required	Allergy to contrast
	Damage to nerves and blood vessels
High success rate	

Mark Scheme for Examiner

	0	1	2	3
Introduction and General Advice				
Introduces self, and washes hands				
Confirms patient's identity with three points of identification				
Explains procedure, identifies concerns and obtains consent				
Positions and exposes patient				
Checks USS and clotting				
Identifies spot marked ascitic drain, percusses to check				
Preparation				
Obtains equipment and checks expiry dates				
Prepares equipment (including clamping connector tubing)				
Washes hands, dons sterile gloves and apron				
Places drape over the patient				
Cleans site in a spiral pattern 3 times				
Inserting the Ascitic Drain				
Injects LA using the 'withdraw and infiltrate' method				
Withdraws straw-coloured aspirate during deep infiltration				
Withdraws needle and syringe				
Pushes catheter into anaesthetised area, until fluid seen, and then advances a further centimetre				
Removes trocar and attaches catheter to the rubber connector tube				
Secures Bonanno catheter to skin and connects to a catheter bag (unclamping the connector tube)				
Finishing				
Disposes of all sharps immediately				
Disposes of equipment and cleans tray				
Removes gloves, and washes hands				
Documents procedure in the patient's notes				
General Points				
Talks to the patient throughout the procedure				
Avoids patient contamination (i.e. NTT)				

0= Not attempted
1= Performed, with room for improvement
2= Adequately performed
3= Performed beyond level expected

Tip Box

Always send the sample pot with the largest volume of ascitic fluid to cytology, especially if you are suspecting malignancy, because the more you send, the higher the diagnostic yield.

STATION 5.9: LUMBAR PUNCTURE

SCENARIO

Mr Water is a 22-year-old university student who presents to the emergency department (ED) with an acute severe headache. Associated symptoms include fever, vomiting and photophobia. On examination you note marked neck stiffness and Kernig's sign is positive. There are no features suggestive of raised intracranial pressure. You strongly suspect bacterial meningitis and after a CT scan is performed, you are asked by your registrar to perform a lumbar puncture (LP) in order to confirm the diagnosis.

OBJECTIVES

• Perform an LP
• Interpret the results

GENERAL ADVICE

• Performing a LP allows the clinician to obtain a sample of cerebrospinal fluid (CSF) from the sub-arachnoid space below the level at which the spinal cord terminates (L1/L2).

- As a junior doctor, you should only perform this procedure following adequate instruction and under close supervision.
- The key contraindication to performing an LP is raised intracranial pressure (ICP) — the combination of which may result in tonsillar herniation (i.e. 'coning').
- A head CT scan is generally performed before performing an LP.

EQUIPMENT CHECKLIST

(Remember to check expiry dates on all equipment (Fig. 5.31).)
- Tray: either single-use, disposable sterilised tray, or a decontaminated plastic tray that is cleaned pre-/post-procedure
- Sterile gloves
- Single-use apron
- Skin-cleansing swabs
- 25-gauge needle
- Two 21-gauge needles
- 10-mL syringe (for LA)
- 10 mL lidocaine 1%
- LP kit:
  - LP needle (typically 22 gauge)
  - Three-way tap
  - Manometer
  - CSF collection tubes (for microbiology and biochemistry, including glucose)

EXPLAINING AN LP TO THE PATIENT

1. A lumbar puncture is a procedure used to obtain a sample of cerebrospinal fluid — a type of body fluid which bathes the brain and spinal cord.
2. It is important to obtain a sample where possible, because analysis of this fluid allows the medical team to ensure the correct diagnosis is made and appropriate treatment is given.

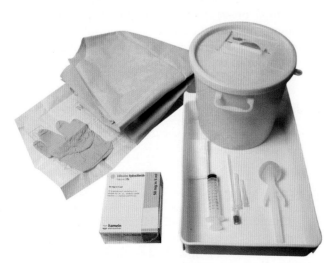

Fig. 5.31 Equipment required to perform an abdominal paracentesis.

3. You will be asked to lie on the bed on your left-hand side with your knees drawn up to your chest and lower back exposed.
4. A needle is inserted into the lower part of the spine where the spinal cord ends, thereby reducing the risk of damage to the cord.
5. An injection of local anaesthetic will be administered first into the skin overlying the puncture site in order to reduce pain. However, you may still experience a sensation of pressure or discomfort.
6. A special needle will then be inserted into the space containing the cerebrospinal fluid and samples of the fluid will be taken.
7. You may experience a headache and nausea following the procedure — these are the most common side effects. You will also need to lie flat for an hour after the procedure.

PERFORMING AN LP

1. Introduce yourself, check the patient's identity and obtain informed consent.
2. Ask the patient to adopt the left lateral position with their lumbar spine exposed.
3. Position the patient with maximal flexion of the spine, hips and knees (widening the intervertebral space).
4. Palpate the superior iliac crest and then follow a vertical line down to the space between the vertebral spines immediately below (corresponding to L3/L4 to L4/L5 intervertebral disc space).
5. Mark this space with an indentation or pen.
6. Wash hands. Put on sterile gloves and single-use apron. Drape the lumbar spine region.
7. Check all of the equipment and open it onto the procedure tray.
8. Sterilise the skin using the swabs.
9. Attach the 21-gauge needle to the 10-mL syringe and draw up the lidocaine.
10. Infiltrate the lidocaine superficially at the marked location using a 25-gauge needle.
11. Exchange the 25-gauge needle for the larger 21-gauge needle and continue to infiltrate lidocaine into the deeper tissues (Note: ensure you aspirate before injecting to reduce the risk of accident intravascular injection).
12. Wait approximately 1 min for the LA to take effect.
13. Take the LP needle and introduce it into the skin at the marked site, with the bevel of the needle pointing up (Fig. 5.32).
14. Carefully advance the needle through the spinal ligaments, feeling a 'give' in resistance as you penetrate the dura mater and enter the subarachnoid space.
15. Now withdraw the stylet from the LP needle and watch for CSF to begin dripping from the needle cuff.

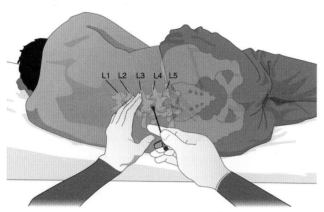

Fig. 5.32 Take time to position the patient correctly before inserting the LP needle (drapes not shown).

16. Attach the manometer and three-way tap to the needle in a vertical position, allowing you to measure CSF pressure (wait for the fluid to stop rising up the column and read off the value).
17. Open the three-way tap and allow 5–10 drops of CSF to drip into each of the three collection tubes (label these tubes 1–3 in the order of collection).
18. If still dripping, collect a glucose sample as well.
19. Reinsert the stylet to stop the flow of CSF and remove the needle.
20. Apply a sterile dressing.

FINISHING

1. Remove the drape, and ensure safe disposal of sharps and packaging.

2. Prescribe simple analgesia when needed for any resultant headache.
3. Label the collection tubes appropriately and send to the lab for:
   • MC&S
   • Cell count
   • Biochemistry (protein and glucose)
4. Document the procedure.
5. Interpret the LP results. A capillary blood sample is also necessary to allow measurement of plasma glucose levels.

DOCUMENT THE PROCEDURE

Document under the following headings:
• LP performed
• Indications for the procedure
• Patient consent
• Relevant laboratory investigations; for example, INR/PT, platelet count
• Procedure technique, sterile preparation, anaesthetic and amount used, amount of fluid obtained, appearance of fluid obtained
• Complications

Present Your Findings

Mr Water, a 22-year-old university student, presented with signs suggestive of bacterial meningitis, therefore an LP was performed. LP results revealed cloudy CSF with a high neutrophil count and protein level of 1.5 g/L and low glucose. The findings are consistent with a diagnosis of bacterial meningitis.

LP Results in Meningitis

	Appearance	Predominant White Cells	Protein (g/L)	Glucose
Normal	Clear	Lymphocytes	0.2–0.4	2/3–0.5 plasma glucose
Viral	Clear	Lymphocytes	0.4–0.8	>0.5 plasma glucose
Bacterial	Turbid	Neutrophils	0.5–2.0	<0.5 plasma glucose
TB	Fibrin web	Lymphocytes	0.5–3.0	<0.5 plasma glucose

Mark Scheme for Examiner

	0	1	2	3
Introduction and General Advice				
Introduces self, and washes hands				
Confirms patient's identity with three points of identification				
Explains procedure, identifies concerns and obtains consent				
Explains common side effects (headache, nausea)				
Checks allergies				
Preparation				
Obtains equipment and checks expiry dates				
Prepares equipment				

Continued

Mark Scheme for Examiner—cont'd

	0	1	2	3
Patient Positioning				
Positions patient in left lateral position with maximal flexion				
Correctly identifies puncture site				
LP				
Washes hands, dons sterile gloves and apron				
Drapes lumbar spine with sterile sheet				
Sterilises skin				
Superficial and deep infiltration of LA				
Waits approximately 1 min for onset of action of LA				
Uses correct technique for LP needle insertion				
Measures CSF pressure using manometer				
Collects CSF sample in collection tubes				
Reinserts stylet and withdraws LP needle				
Safely disposes of needle in sharps bin				
Applies sterile dressing				
Finishing				
Disposes of all sharps immediately				
Removes drape, apron and gloves and disposes of them in clinical waste bin				
Removes gloves, and washes hands				
Labels collection tubes at the bedside				
Documents procedure in the patient notes				
General Points				
Talks to the patient throughout the procedure				
Avoids patient contamination (i.e. NTT)				

0= Not attempted
1= Performed, with room for improvement
2= Adequately performed
3= Performed beyond level expected

QUESTIONS AND ANSWERS FOR CANDIDATE

What are the key contraindications to performing a LP?

- Raised ICP
- Coagulopathy or low platelet count
- Cutaneous infection at the LP site

What clinical features are suggestive of raised ICP?

- Papilloedema
- Focal neurological signs
- Decreased level of consciousness (Glasgow Coma Scale (GCS) <8/15)
- Bradycardia, hypertension and an irregular breathing pattern (Cushing's triad)

In what type of meningitis would you expect to find an increased neutrophil count?

- Bacterial meningitis

Tip Box

When introducing the LP needle, imagine you are aiming for the umbilicus — this will help to ensure correct positioning. Many doctors will tell you that this practical skill involves a certain amount of 'feel' — practise makes perfect!

Fact Box

The anatomical layers that are penetrated when inserting an LP needle are (Fig. 5.33):
1. Skin
2. Supraspinous ligament
3. Interspinous ligament and ligamentum flavum
4. (Extradural space)
5. Dura mater
6. Arachnoid mater

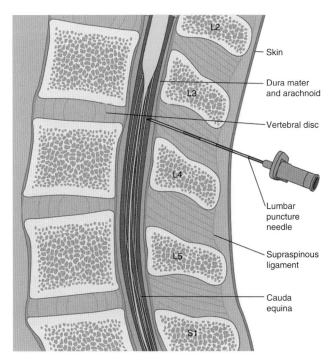

Fig. 5.33 The key layers penetrated when inserting an LP needle.

STATION 5.10: PROCTOSCOPY

SCENARIO

Mr Walker is a 68-year-old man who presents to his GP with constipation. He has also noticed bright red blood on the toilet paper and feels that his back passage has been itchy over the last few months. Prolapsed haemorrhoids were visible on inspection. Please perform proctoscopy on this patient to investigate further the cause of his signs and symptoms.

OBJECTIVES

- To learn how to perform proctoscopy

GENERAL ADVICE

- Proctoscopy also involves a digital rectal examination beforehand. The patient should be advised that the procedure may be uncomfortable at times but should not be painful.
- Check the type of proctoscope being used during the examination. Plastic proctoscopes are typically disposable whereas metal proctoscopes can be reused if sterilised. Some proctoscopes also allow an attachment of a light source to allow better visualisation of the rectal mucosa.

EQUIPMENT CHECKLIST

(Remember to check expiry dates on all equipment.)
- Room with curtain around the examination bed
- Three water-soluble lubricating gel sachets
- Paper towels
- Proctoscope with fitting obturator (helps to guide the proctoscope in)
- Light source (either attachable to the proctoscope or a movable lamp)
- Two pairs of non-sterile gloves

EXPLAINING PROCTOSCOPY TO THE PATIENT

1. Proctoscopy is done to identify the presence of diseases in the back passage. It is also used to investigate for causes of rectal bleeding and to monitor the growth of any polyps or cancers that may be present.
2. The doctor may ask you to have an enema before the procedure. This is a liquid that is put into the back passage to empty your bowel before your procedure.
3. The doctor will typically examine your back passage using a gloved finger first and then use a lubricated proctoscope to examine your rectum.
4. Some patients feel pressure, cramping, fullness or the need to pass stool during this examination. It is also not unusual to pass wind during the procedure.
5. Sometimes the doctor may use additional instruments to take samples of tissue for further testing.

PERFORMING PROCTOSCOPY

PREPARATION

1. Introduce yourself to the patient and obtain consent.
2. Ask the patient if they would like a chaperone present during this examination. If the patient declies, ensure that you document this in the notes.
3. Obtain the equipment.
4. Ask the patient to expose the body below the waist and to lie in the left lateral decubitus position.
5. Ask the patient to have their buttocks at the edge of the bed with their legs flexed at 90 degrees.
6. Don two pairs of non-sterile gloves.
7. Inspect the perianal area and anus visually for any abnormalities.
8. Lubricate the index finger of your dominant hand, and rest the open packet of lubricant on a paper towel.
9. Warn the patient that you are about to examine their back passage using your finger first and that they may feel uncomfortable.
10. Perform a digital rectal examination, testing the rectum for the presence of any masses and pain.
11. Ask the patient to 'bear down' on your finger to assess sphincter tone.
12. Withdraw your finger slowly to avoid sudden spasm, and look at your glove for any blood or stool.
13. Remove the outer gloves and discard then into a nearby bin.

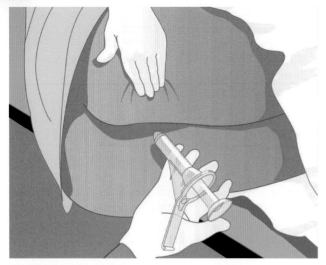

Fig. 5.34 Warn the patient before inserting the proctoscope.

14. Fully introduce the obturator into the proctoscope and lubricate both generously.
15. Hold the proctoscope in a position that maintains pressure on the obturator, keeping it held into the proctoscope.
16. Separate the buttocks with your non-dominant hand, either using your forefinger and thumb or lifting the top buttock with your hand.
17. Warn the patient that you are about to examine their back passage using the proctoscope and then introduce the proctoscope gently into the rectum. Aim the proctoscope towards the umbilicus initially and then towards the sacrum (Fig. 5.34).
18. Remove the obturator once the proctoscope has been fully inserted (Fig. 5.35).
19. Attach the light source (if required) (Fig. 5.36).
20. Inspect for mucosal abnormalities.

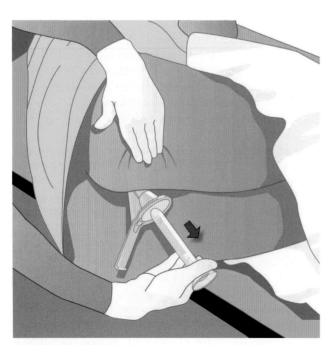

Fig. 5.35 Removing the obturator.

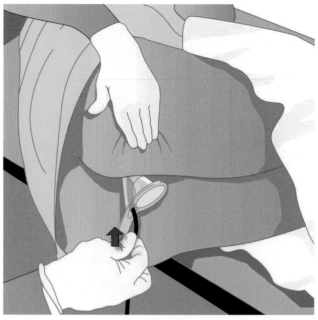

Fig. 5.36 A light source can be attached if required.

21. Once examination is complete, ask the patient to strain down gently on the proctoscope whilst you slowly withdraw the device.
22. Look again for haemorrhoids and significant rectal prolapse.
23. Wipe the perineum for any residual lubricant or stool and when you withdraw, put the curtain around, allowing the patient to get dressed with privacy.

DOCUMENT THE PROCEDURE

Document under the following headings:
• Digital rectal examination and proctoscopy performed
• Indications for the procedure
• Patient consent and presence/absence of chaperone
• Signs on external inspection
• Rectal examination:
  • Any masses or stool on the glove on withdrawal
  • Whether the patient experienced any pain
• Proctoscopy:
  • Any abnormalities detected
  • Whether the patient experienced any pain
• Complications
• Subsequent tests ordered, if any

Present Your Findings

Mr Walker is a 68-year-old man who presented to his general practioner (GP) with constipation, itching and rectal bleeding. Inspection revealed prolapsed haemorrhoids, digital rectal examination demonstrated bright red blood on the glove and proctoscopy also confirmed haemorrhoids. I would refer him for further investigations to exclude other causes of bleeding; these may involve sigmoidoscopy and biopsy. At this time, banding of haemorrhoids could be performed if no other cause of rectal bleeding was detected.

Features to Assess

On Perianal Inspection	On Digital Rectal Examination	On Proctoscopy
• Anal fissures • Ulcers • Warts • Skin tags • Pilonidal abscesses • Perianal fistulae • Signs of incontinence • Visible rectal prolapse • Haemorrhoids • Pus	• Rectal masses • Polyps • Abscesses • Haemorrhoids • Prostatic enlargement • Sphincter tone	• Haemorrhoids • Rectal polyps • Warts • Fissures • Rectal prolapse • Mucosal inflammation (suggesting Crohn's disease or ulcerative colitis) • Rectal cancer

Mark Scheme for Examiner

	0	1	2	3
Introduction and General Advice				
Introduces self, and washes hands				
Confirms patient's identity with three points of identification				
Explains procedure, identifies concerns and obtains consent				
Offers chaperone (documents in notes)				
Positions and exposes patient				
Preparation				
Obtains equipment and checks expiry dates				
Washes hands, dons two pairs of non-sterile gloves				
Inspects perianal area and anus				
Performs digital rectal examination				
Performing Proctoscopy				
Removes outer gloves. Lubricates proctoscope				
Separates patient's buttocks				
Maintains pressure on the obturator				
Introduces proctoscope				
Removes obturator after complete insertion				
Attaches light source and inspects mucosa				
Withdraws proctoscope				
Inspects perianal area again				
Finishing				
Wipes excess lubricant and covers patient				
Removes gloves, and washes hands				
Documents procedure in the patient's notes				
General Points				
Talks to the patient throughout the procedure				
Avoids patient contamination (i.e. NTT)				

0= Not attempted
1= Performed, with room for improvement
2= Adequately performed
3= Performed beyond level expected

❓ QUESTIONS AND ANSWERS FOR CANDIDATE

Name the types of scopes used to investigate the lower gastrointestinal tract.
• Proctoscope
• Rigid sigmoidoscopy
• Flexible sigmoidoscopy

Name three possible signs of sexual assault on inspection of the perianal and anal region.
• Reflex anal dilatation
• Venous congestion
• Anal fissures
• Anal laxity

- Anal fold changes
- Swelling
- Erythema

What are haemorrhoids and how are they treated?
- Haemorrhoids are also known as piles.
- They are swollen veins in the lowest part of the rectum and anus.
- They can be managed conservatively (warm bath, cold compression), medically (ointments or suppositories, stool softeners) or surgically (rubber band ligation, cauterisation, haemorrhoidectomy).

In the assessment of adult victims of sexual violence, under what circumstances is proctoscopy warranted?
- Only in cases of postassault anal bleeding, severe anal pain, or if there is suspicion of the presence of a foreign body inside the rectum

 Tip Box

If anal spasm occurs during rectal examination, ask the patient to breathe in deeply, then out and relax. Anal fissures are one source of pain and spasms. The use of LA gel may help.

 Fact Box

If there is any clinical suspicion of sexual assault, it would be wise to defer the examination until a forensic expert is present to collect specimens or other evidence. It may also be advisable to contact the clinical lead for child protection if the patient is 18 years or younger. Swabs should be taken for *Chlamydia* and other sexually transmitted infections if clinically suspected.

STATION 5.11: INSTRUMENTS

SCENARIO

On this table are a number of instruments. Please take one and tell the examiner what you know about it.

OBJECTIVE

- To be able to recognise and discuss common medical instruments.

GENERAL ADVICE

- If you are given a choice, it might help to pick first the instrument that you are most familiar with. This will help you to gain confidence and momentum before you approach more difficult items.
- Take the item and hold it delicately and securely in your hands. To demonstrate familiarity to the examiner, try holding the instrument in the position that you would use in practice. Make a mental image of the instrument, then turn to the examiner and try not to look back at your hands.
- Keep a mental note to stop talking when you feel you have covered your framework for this station. Try not to give opinions and details you are unsure about.
- Above all, speak with a measured pace and confidence.
- The following structure can be applied to almost any instrument and will give you a framework for your answer:
  - Name and type of instrument
  - Indications for use or real scenario of where you have seen it used
  - How it is used
  - Complications of using said instrument
  - Contraindications

COMMON INSTRUMENTS

OROPHARYNGEAL (OP) AIRWAY (FIG. 5.37)

1. This is an OP airway, also known as a Guedel airway. It is an example of a non-definitive airway adjunct.
2. This device helps maintain a patent airway in unconscious patients to facilitate oxygenation and ventilation. It is used widely in anaesthetics and on patients in the ED with an impaired conscious level.

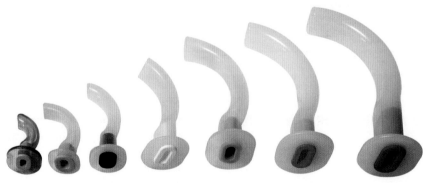

Fig. 5.37 Ensure you are familiar with all airway adjuncts.

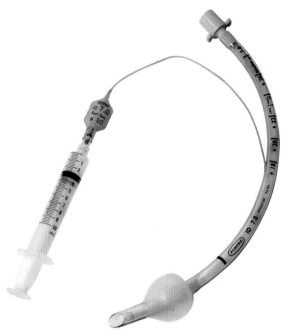

Fig. 5.38 ET tube.

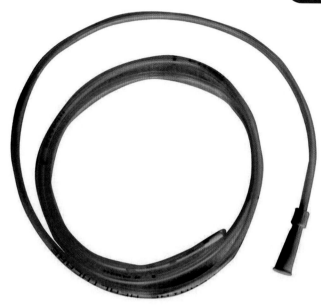

Fig. 5.39 NG tube.

3. The correct size is chosen by measuring the distance from the incisors to the angle of the mandible. It is then held with two forefingers and a thumb at the thick plastic attached to the oval disc. During insertion the Guedel airway is held in a position where the spout points towards the operator, and the bend in the device points away from the operator. The Guedel airway is then inserted into the oral cavity using the bend in the device to push the tongue back. The device is rotated 180 degrees as it descends past the hard palate. This approach reduces the risk of pushing the tongue backwards.
4. Complications of using a Guedel airway include:
   • Trauma to the oropharynx
   • Upper-airway obstruction
   • Stimulation of the gag reflex, resulting in vomiting
5. Main contraindications include:
   • Active airway reflexes (typically in conscious patients)
   • Active bleeding

ENDOTRACHEAL (ET) TUBE (FIG. 5.38)

1. This is a cuffed ET tube and is an example of a definitive airway.
2. This device is used in anaesthetics and in intensive care during the intubation and ventilation of unconscious patients.
3. This device needs to be inserted by a trained health professional in a controlled environment. It is inserted into the trachea under direct vision with the use of a laryngoscope to identify the glottis after insertion, the balloon cuff is inflated with the use of

a syringe to keep the tube in place and prevent aspiration of gastric contents into the respiratory tract.
4. Tube complications include:
   • Misplacement of the tube into the oesophagus and descent of the tube into a main bronchus (commonly the right main bronchus)
   • Impaction of the tube against the airway
   • Dental/lip/gum trauma
   • Pulmonary aspiration of gastric contents
   • Oesophageal or tracheal perforation
   • Subglottic stenosis
   • Vocal cord paralysis
5. A relative contraindication to intubation includes:
   • Cervical spine injury, where immobilisation makes intubation difficult
   • Severe airway trauma or obstruction, where an emergency cricothyrotomy is likely to be more useful

NASOGASTRIC TUBE (NG) (FIG. 5.39)

1. This is an NG tube, of which there are two types: Fine- and wide-bore.
2. Fine-bore tubes are used for enteral feeding in patients on the ward with an unsafe swallow assessment, and also following gastrointestinal surgery. Wide-bore tubes are typically used to provide gastric decompression in patients with bowel obstruction or following elective upper gastrointestinal surgery.
3. The distance required to insert the tube is sized by measuring the distance of the tube from the nostril to the xiphisternum passing via the tragus of the ear. The lower 10 cm is then lubricated and advanced along the base of the nasal cavity in an upright patient. The patient is asked to sip water using a straw when the tube reaches the posterior

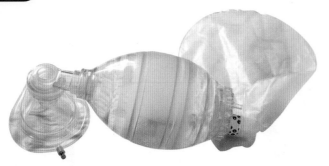

Fig. 5.40 Bag valve mask.

pharynx. This manoeuvre aids the introduction of the tube into the oesophagus. The tube is inserted to the sized distance and then a little more to ensure correct positioning, which is confirmed via testing aspirates with pH paper and chest X-ray.

4. The most common complications are:
   - Damage to the nasal turbinates (resulting in bleeding) during insertion
   - Misplacements, e.g. into the trachea
5. NG tubes are contraindicated in:
   - Base-of-skull fractures
   - Severe mid-face trauma
   - Recent nasal surgery
6. Relative contraindications include:
   - Oesophageal varices
   - Obstructed oesophagus
   - Coagulation abnormalities

BAG VALVE MASK (FIG. 5.40)

1. This is a bag valve mask used to provide positive-pressure ventilation.
2. This is used to oxygenate and ventilate patients who are not breathing or are breathing inadequately. This device is frequently used in anaesthetics and in the acute care of patients until a more definitive airway is implemented.
3. The bag valve mask can be connected to an oxygen port on the wall to provide concentrated oxygen but also works independently and is self-filling. The mask is triangular in shape, and its tip should be placed just over the bridge of the patient's nose. The larger portion of the mask should be placed between the lower lips and the chin to provide a good seal. Although one person can operate this device, it is more comfortable with two, where one person places the mask firmly on the patient's face whilst simultaneously providing a jaw-thrust, and the other squeezes the bag.
4. Complications of a bag valve mask include:
   - Aspiration
   - Hypo-/hyperventilation
5. Bag valve mask ventilation is relatively contraindicated:
   - After paralysis and induction, due to the increased risk of aspiration

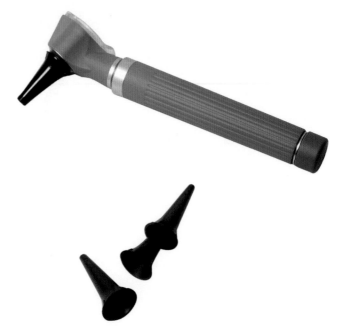

Fig. 5.41 Otoscope.

6. You must use it with care in patients with suspected cervical spine trauma or facial fractures.

OTOSCOPE (FIG. 5.41)

1. This device is an otoscope and there are four main types: direct, indirect, pneumatic and operating. The standard direct otoscope can be either wall-mounted or battery-operated. The device can additionally be attached to different-sized speculums.
2. It is used by doctors to examine the external auditory canal and tympanic membrane for outer- and middle-ear pathology.
3. The direct otoscope is typically held in the same hand as the side of the ear being examined. It is held the same way as a pen, with the fingers placed on its neck next to the eyepiece and with the speculum facing away from the operator. After activating the light source and inspecting the external auditory canal and surrounding areas, the pinna is manually retracted superiorly and posteriorly with the other hand. The otoscope is gently introduced into the ear canal with the clinician's little finger extended and rested on the patient to provide stability to the instrument.
4. Complications are rare but mainly include trauma to the ear canal.

◎ Common Instruments

Here is a list of other common equipment that it will be useful to look up

LINES
- Central venous line
- Hickman line
- Swan–Ganz catheter

Common Instruments—cont'd

FLUIDS
Crystalloids
- Hartmann's solution
- 0.9% saline
- Dextrose saline

Colloids
- Gelofusin
- Albumin
- Blood products

COLORECTAL
- Rigid sigmoidoscope
- Flexible sigmoidoscope
- Gabriel syringe
- Laparoscopic ports

ORTHOPAEDICS
- Knee prostheses
- Hip prostheses
- Dynamic hip screw
- Medullary nail

AIRWAYS
- Nasopharyngeal airway
- Laryngeal mask airway
- Tracheostomy tube

Where are the defibrillator pads placed on a person?
- One pad is placed over the left precordium at the lower part of the chest, and the second typically below the right clavicle. If the patient has a pacemaker, you would place the pads at least 8 cm away.

How many litres of oxygen do you connect to nasal cannulae?
- A nasal cannula is typically used to carry 2–4 L/min of oxygen to the patient. Using flow rates above 5 L can cause discomfort to the patient as the flow becomes turbulent.

Name two limitations of using pH testing to verify NG tube position.
- Stomach pH can be affected by medications.
- Stomach pH can be affected by the frequency of feeds.
- It may be difficult to obtain aspirate from the NG tube.

What are the typical daily fluid and electrolyte requirements for maintenance of the average adult who is nil by mouth?
- 25–30 ml/kg/24 h of water
- 1 mmol/kg/24 h of sodium, potassium and chloride individually
- 5–100 g/24 h of glucose

Mark Scheme for Examiner

	0	1	2	3
Introduction				
Introduces self, and washes hands				
Identifies name of equipment				
Describes main indications for use				
Outlines complications				
Outlines contraindications				
Practical Skills				
Holds equipment in correct position				
Simulates use of equipment on mannequin correctly				
General Points				
Speaks clearly with a measured pace				
Demonstrates confidence with equipment use				
Answers questions on equipment				

0= Not attempted
1= Performed, with room for improvement
2= Adequately performed
3= Performed beyond level expected

❓ QUESTIONS AND ANSWERS FOR CANDIDATE

What device can be used to provide rescue breaths safely during cardiopulmonary resuscitation?
- A pocket face mask is often used and contains an attachable one-way valve to protect the operator from infectious bodily fluids such as vomit.

Tip Box

When you are next in surgery, try to ask a member of staff politely to go through the names of the instruments on the table with you. It makes it easier to remember when you are looking at real objects compared to looking at images.

Fact Box

Flexible sigmoidoscopy provides more patient comfort and diagnostic value and is easier for carrying out procedures like biopsy compared to rigid sigmoidoscopy.

STATION 5.12: SUTURING

SCENARIO

Mr Harrison, a 27-year-old man, has presented to the ED with a wound to his forearm. Please suture the wound together using a simple technique.

OBJECTIVE

- To perform basic suturing

GENERAL ADVICE

- Start this station by assessing the wound to see if it requires referral to senior or specialist surgical colleagues.
- It is important to check the neurovascular supply to the region and involve senior staff where wounds involve tendons, nerves or large vessels.
- It may be useful to order an X-ray where retained or deep foreign bodies are suspected.
- A plastic surgery referral is essential for complex facial lacerations, especially those involving the vermilion line (the border between the lips and skin).

EQUIPMENT CHECKLIST

(Remember to check expiry dates on all equipment.)
- An assistant
- Iodine solution
- Sterile water
- Gauze
- Needle holder
- Toothed forceps
- Scissors
- Suture(s): for example, 4/0 synthetic, non-absorbable monofilament with a curved needle
- Lidocaine with 1/200,000 adrenaline (to minimise bleeding, but do not use adrenaline on extremities due to vasoconstrictive effect)
- 5-mL syringe
- 21-gauge needle
- 25-gauge needle to administer
- Equipment trolley
- Sharps bin: the sharps bin should always be taken to the point of care
- Sterile gloves
- Sterile dressing

Note: A lot of this equipment may come in a pre-formed 'sterile pack' for suturing.

EXPLAINING SUTURING TO THE PATIENT

1. Suturing is a technique used to close up wounds using a needle attached to thread.
2. Before starting, the wound will be cleaned and a numbing agent will be injected around the cut for pain relief.
3. The wound will then be closed up with sutures and a bandage applied over the area.
4. Your wound will be inspected at a later date, and the sutures may be removed when the wound has healed.
5. It is important to inform the doctor if the wound looks infected or continues to bleed considerably after discharge.

SUTURING

PROCEDURE PREPARATION

1. Introduce yourself to the patient and obtain consent.
2. Obtain equipment, wash hands and don sterile gloves using the aseptic technique (Fig. 5.42).
3. Assemble the suturing equipment on a sterile field on the equipment trolley.
4. Withdraw lidocaine into a 5-mL syringe via a 21-gauge needle.
5. Detach the needle without resheathing, and discard it in a sharps bin.
6. Attach a 25-gauge needle with its sheath on, and place the needle and syringe into the needle's packet.

WOUND PREPARATION

1. Remove large, visible debris from the wound using forceps.
2. Use sterile water to soak gauze and clean the wound gently.

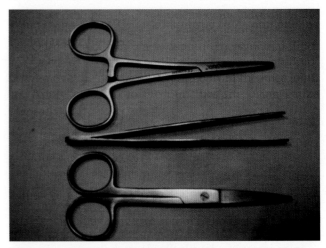
Fig. 5.42 (From top to bottom) Needle holder, forceps and scissors.

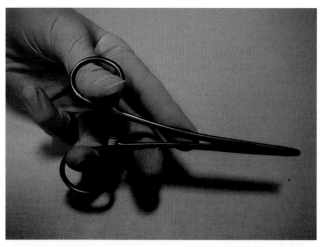

Fig. 5.43 Holding the needle holder.

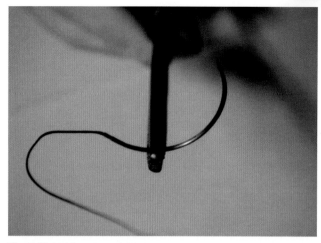

Fig. 5.45 Holding the needle.

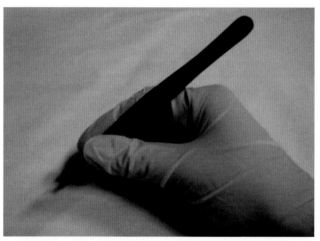

Fig. 5.44 Holding the forceps.

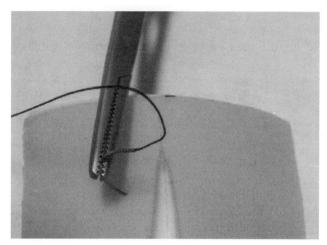

Fig. 5.46 Inserting the needle.

3. Administer LA into the skin and soft tissues around the wound in a circular pattern via the 'aspirate and infiltrate' method.
4. Soak iodine solution on gauze and clean the wound.
5. Dry the wound with a clean gauze.

SUTURING
(BASIC INTERRUPTED SUTURING TECHNIQUE)

1. Hold the needle holder in your dominant hand with your thumb and ring finger (Fig. 5.43).
2. Hold the toothed forceps in your other hand using a pen grip (Fig. 5.44).
3. Remove the needle and suture from the packaging with the needle holder, and reposition the needle using the forceps (Fig. 5.45).
4. Bring your thumb and ring finger together to lock the needle into the needle holder; several clicks should be heard.
5. The first suture should be in the centre of the wound.
6. With the forceps, gently manipulate the wound's edge.

7. Insert the needle perpendicular to the skin's surface approximately 5 mm from the wound edge (Fig. 5.46).
8. Advance the needle through the wound in a circular arc, aiming to exit in the middle of the wound.
9. Grasp the needle with the forceps, taking care not to blunt the tip of the needle.
10. Release the needle from the needle holder.
11. Withdraw the needle with the forceps and regrip with the needle holder.
12. Use the forceps as a pulley to leave approximately 4 cm of thread at the original insertion site.
13. Reinsert the needle from within the wound and aim to exit about 5 mm from the wound edge (Fig. 5.47).
14. Once again, grasp the needle with the forceps, release from needle holder and withdraw the needle to pull the thread taut.

TYING A SURGICAL KNOT

1. Place the needle holder in between the two ends of the suture thread, forming a 'V' (Fig. 5.48).

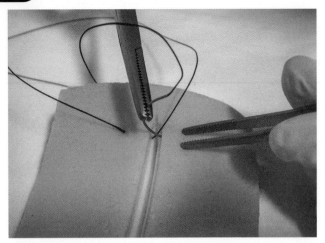

Fig. 5.47 Reinserting the needle on the opposite side.

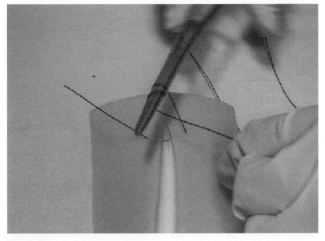

Fig. 5.49 Looping the suture.

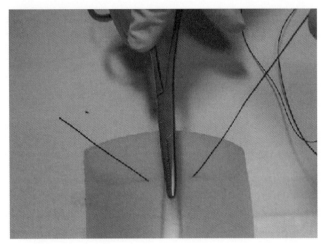

Fig. 5.48 The first 'V'.

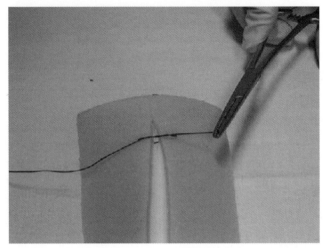

Fig. 5.50 The first knot.

2. Loop the thread attached to the needle around the needle holder 3 times in a clockwise fashion (Fig. 5.49). Keep hold of this long end of the suture.
3. Grasp the very tip of the short end of the suture (from the original insertion site) with the needle holder. Pull the two ends of sutures in opposite directions at right angles to the wound, forming the first knot (Fig. 5.50).
4. Form a 'V' shape with the two ends of the sutures (Fig. 5.51). Then place the needle holder in between the two ends.
5. Loop the thread attached to the needle around the needle holder twice in an anticlockwise fashion (Fig. 5.52). Grasp the very tip of the short end of the suture with the needle holder. Pull the two ends of the suture in opposite directions at right angles to the wound. This is the second knot.
6. Follow steps 1–3 above to lay down the third knot.
7. Reposition your knots so that they are not lying over the line of the wound (Fig. 5.53).
8. Cut the ends of the suture, leaving approximately 5 mm each end (Fig. 5.54). Ensure the suture needle is immediately disposed of in a sharps bin.

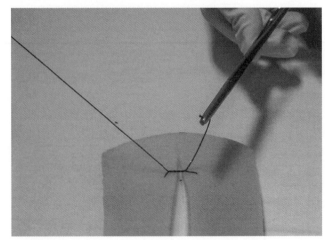

Fig. 5.51 The second 'V'.

9. Repeat steps 1–8 above 5–10 mm on both sides along from your first suture (Fig. 5.55).
10. Ensure that all the wound edges are successfully brought together.

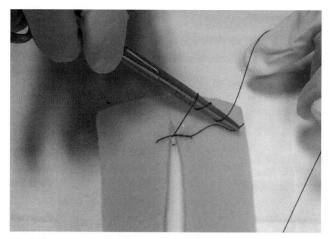

Fig. 5.52 Looping the suture for the second knot.

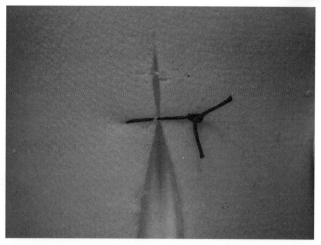

Fig. 5.54 An uninterrupted suture.

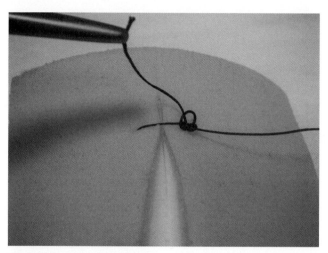

Fig. 5.53 Reposition your knot.

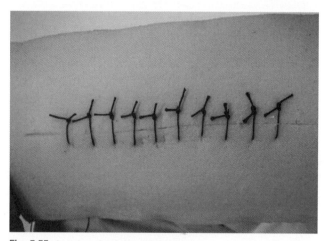

Fig. 5.55 A series of uninterrupted sutures.

DOCUMENT THE PROCEDURE

Document under the following headings:
- Details of site of laceration and wound assessment
- Any referrals made
- Amount of LA used
- Wound suturing performed on patient
- Complications
- Estimated blood loss
- Details of follow-up and wound aftercare

WOUND AFTERCARE

- Apply a dressing over the wound if required.
- Always administer a tetanus booster if the patient has not had one in the past 10 years or if the wound is contaminated.
- Advise the patient to keep the wound dry whilst showering and washing.
- Educate the patient on signs of wound infection (for example, redness, soreness, discharge), and advise them to seek medical help if this occurs.

❓ QUESTIONS AND ANSWERS FOR CANDIDATE

Name some alternatives to suturing.
- Steri-Strips
- Staples
- Tissue adhesives (glue)

When are non-absorbable sutures removed?
- Sutures will normally be removed in 7–14 days (4–5 days in the case of the face).
- This can usually be done with the agreement of their GP or district nurse.

When is a mattress suture indicated?
When the skin edges are difficult to evert. They provide good dermis-to-dermis contact and can be used in conjunction with simple interrupted sutures. When a wound is not holding together; for example, if the wound edges are under tension.

Name two risk factors for wound infections that may indicate prophylactic antibiotics.
- Presence of a foreign body
- Heavily soiled wounds

Mark Scheme for Examiner

	0	1	2	3
Introduction and General Advice				
Introduces self, and washes hands				
Confirms patient's identity with three points of identification				
Explains procedure, identifies concerns and obtains consent				
Checks allergies				
Inspects and assesses wound site				
Discusses referral to specialist surgeons if appropriate				
Preparation				
Obtains equipment and checks expiry dates				
Washes hands, dons sterile gloves				
Injects LA using the 'withdraw and infiltrate' method				
Cleans wound site with sterile water and iodine solution				
Suturing				
Inserts needle perpendicular to skin at correct distance				
Withdraws needle with forceps from the centre of the wound				
Re-enters wound parallel to original insertion				
Pulls suture threat taut with forceps				
Ties three knots for each suture and repositions knot				
Ensures wound edges are successfully brought together				
Finishing				
Places dressing over wound				
Disposes of all sharps immediately				
Disposes of equipment				
Removes gloves, and wash hands				
Documents procedure in the patient's notes				
General Points				
Talks to the patient throughout the procedure				
Avoids patient contamination (i.e. NTT)				

0= Not attempted
1= Performed, with room for improvement
2= Adequately performed
3= Performed beyond level expected

- Bites (including human bites)
- Puncture wounds
- Open fractures

What is the maximum dose of lidocaine that can be administered for use as LA?

- 3 mg/kg of lidocaine without adrenaline, 7 mg/kg of lidocaine with adrenaline

 Tip Box

Use the forceps to grip the needle with the needle holder. Never handle the needle with your fingers.

 Fact Box

Vertical mattress sutures are particularly useful in wounds under tension, and where the skin is prone to naturally inverting into the wounds.

STATION 5.13: SURGICAL GOWNING AND GLOVING

SCENARIO

You have been asked to assist in surgery. Scrub up using an aseptic technique.

OBJECTIVES

- Scrub up aseptically
- Maintain a sterile field

GENERAL ADVICE

- Always ask if you are unsure about touching objects in the operating theatre. This will help maintain sterility.

- It is important not to touch sterile gowns or gloves when opening their packets as this results in contamination.
- The accepted clothing underneath a surgical gown is surgical scrubs with comfortable theatre shoes, and these should not be worn outside the hospital.
- Nails should be short and without nail polish.
- Rings, watches, jewellery, wallets and mobile phones should be locked away out of the operating theatre.

EQUIPMENT CHECKLIST (FIG. 5.56)

- An assistant
- Surgical cap
- Face mask ± eye shield
- Theatre shoes or boots
- Sink with elbow tap handles and elbow-activated antiseptic wash
- Sterile paper towels
- Hand scrubber packet (including brush and sponge)
- Gowning trolley
- Correctly sized sterile gown
- Correctly sized sterile gloves

SCRUBBING-UP PROCEDURES

NON-STERILE PROCEDURES

1. Wear a surgical cap before entering the surgical scrubbing room. This should be tied so that any falling hair is trapped in the cap. Put on theatre shoes.
2. Wash hands at the sink inside the scrubbing room, and dry them with paper towels nearby.
3. Tie on a face mask ± eye shield (depending on the type of surgery), ensuring that it covers both mouth and nose (Fig. 5.57).
4. Find the gowning trolley and obtain the sterile gown. Do not collect the gloves yet.

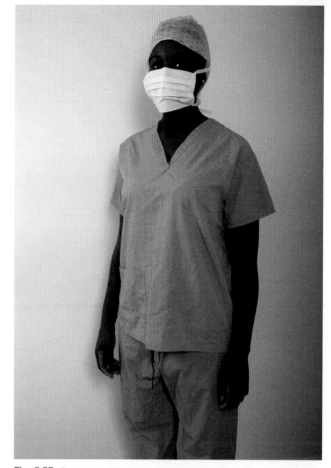

Fig. 5.57 Correct position for face mask.

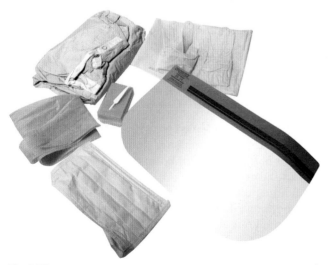

Fig. 5.56 Open all equipment you require before starting to scrub.

5. Open the packet containing the surgical gown in an aseptic fashion, and gently drop it facing upwards on the gowning trolley.
6. Opening the packet should reveal a surgical gown below sterile paper towels. Obtain the hand scrubber packet.
7. Open a packet of sterile gloves (of the appropriate size), placing them so that you still have access to the sterile paper towels.

FIRST WASH TECHNIQUE

1. Open the tap to get the water flowing at a comfortable temperature and rate which avoids splashing. *You must not touch the taps with your hands after this step.*
2. Wet hands up to the elbows, ensuring that water is flowing from the fingers down to the elbows throughout the procedure (Fig. 5.58).
3. Open the hand scrubber packet and use the pick inside to remove any dirt or debris from under the nails, then discard the pick into a nearby bin.
4. Press the lever of the antiseptic bottle with the elbow of one arm whilst positioning the hand of the other arm under the bottle to receive the solution onto the sponge part of the scrubber.

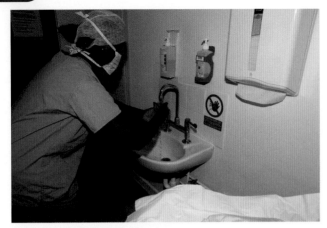

Fig. 5.58 Wash hands up to the elbows.

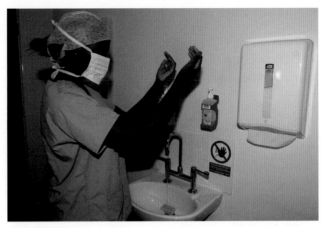

Fig. 5.60 Remember that you are now sterile and should avoid any contamination.

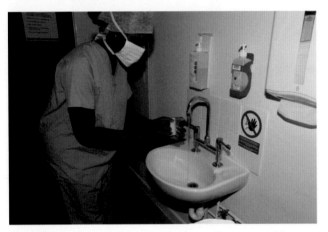

Fig. 5.59 Use the sponge to clean the fingernails more carefully.

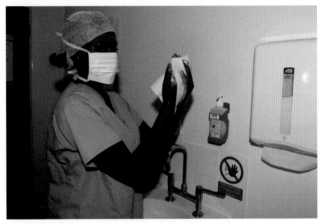

Fig. 5.61 Always start drying from the hands.

5. Use the sponge to clean the fingernails, palms, back of hands, wrists and forearms thoroughly and work downwards to the elbows (Fig. 5.59).
6. Discard the sponge into a nearby bin, and then wash the hands up to the elbows.

SECOND WASH TECHNIQUE

1. Press the lever of the antiseptic bottle with the elbow of one arm whilst positioning the hand of the other arm under the bottle to receive the solution on to the other hand.
2. Wash hands according to the World Health Organization (WHO) guidelines (Station 8.1).
3. Rotationally rub the wrist, working down to the elbows with one hand, and vice versa.
4. Wash the hands up to the elbows in a 'swinging motion'.

THIRD WASH TECHNIQUE

1. Perform exactly the same wash for both arms but stop two-thirds down the forearm, not reaching the elbows.

2. Place your arms bent at the elbow in front of you and allow the water to drip off your elbows (Fig. 5.60).
3. Close the tap with your elbow, taking care to minimise contact as much as possible.
4. Return to the gowning trolley and use one paper towel per arm, drying from fingertips to elbows in a dabbing motion. *Do not go back and dry in the opposite direction.* Discard the paper towel once used and repeat for the other arm (Figs 5.61 and 5.62).

SCRUBBING UP

1. Arrange your hands so your fingers are close together and thumbs are pointing upwards. Place each hand in the arm holes of the gown (Fig. 5.63).
2. Lift the gown.
3. Holding the gown gently but firmly, step back from the trolley, ensuring there is no equipment nearby.
4. Extend your elbows from your body and move your arms apart. The gown should open itself and you will be able to slip your hands and arms in the gown (Fig. 5.64).

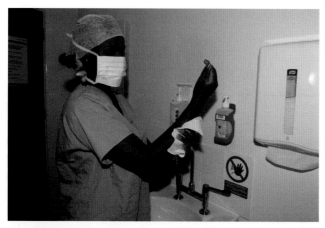

Fig. 5.62 Always start drying from the hands.

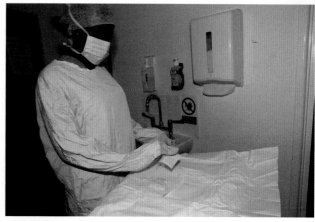

Fig. 5.65 Putting on sterile gloves, correct preparation.

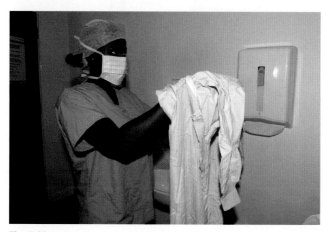

Fig. 5.63 Remember that the gown is also sterile and should not touch any surface.

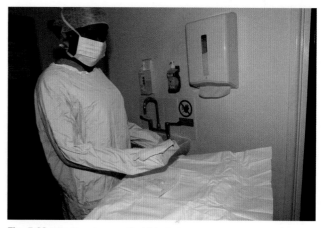

Fig. 5.66 Flip the glove so that it is facing you.

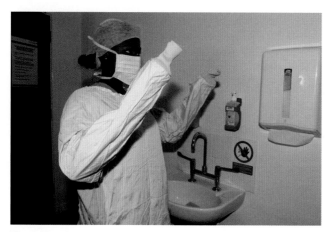

Fig. 5.64 Straighten your arms.

5. Do not let your hands go beyond the cuff.
6. Ask an assistant to fasten your neck collar and tie at the back.

DONNING GLOVES USING THE 'CLOSED GLOVE TECHNIQUE'

1. Gripping through the gown cuffs, place the glove packet upside down.

2. Unfold the packet by gripping its edges. The right glove should now be on the left and the left glove on the right.
3. Grasp the folded cuff of the right glove with the right hand (Fig. 5.65).
4. Pick the right glove up and rest it on your right hand. The fingers of the glove should be pointing towards your body, the palm should be facing outwards and the thumb should not be visible as it is resting on your hand (Fig. 5.66).
5. Whilst keeping your grip on the folded cuff with your right hand, use your left hand (through the gown's cuff) to grab the other folded cuff, which is facing you (Fig. 5.67).
6. Bring the cuff of the glove facing you over the fingers of your right hand and slide your right hand into the glove (Fig. 5.68).
7. Unroll the rest of the glove to allow it to fit more securely and comfortably on your right hand. Then straighten the gown so the cuffs cover a little more than your wrist (Fig. 5.69).
8. Follow the steps above for the left hand.

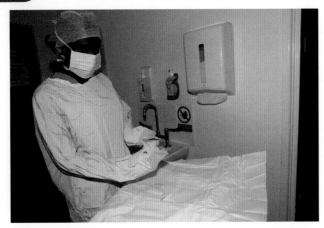

Fig. 5.67 Grip the glove.

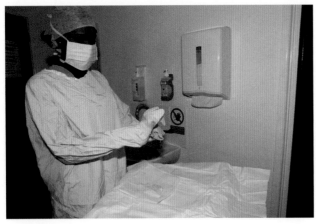

Fig. 5.68 Slide your hand in the glove.

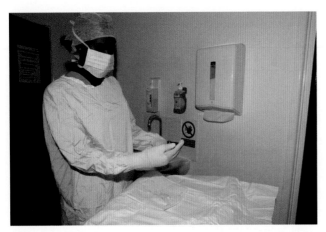

Fig. 5.69 Now position the glove.

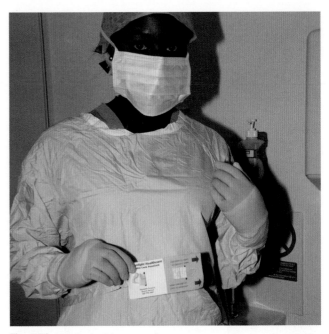

Fig. 5.70 This is the 'dance card'.

SECURING THE GOWN

1. Find the piece of card with two ties attached. This is called the 'dance card' (Fig. 5.70).
2. Hold onto the short tie with your left hand and remove it from the gown. Do not let go of the short tie.
3. Give the 'dance card' with the right tie attached to the assistant, ensuring that there is no hand contact (Fig. 5.71).
4. Let go of the 'dance card' and turn 360 degrees anti-clockwise (Fig. 5.72).
5. Grip the tie and pull away from the card held by the assistant.
6. Tie a simple reef knot with the ties in your left and right hand (Fig. 5.73).
7. Keep your hands near your chest to ensure you remain sterile (Fig. 5.74).

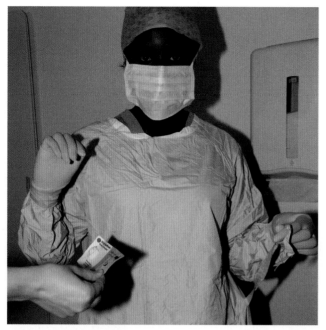

Fig. 5.71 Hand the 'dance card' to assistant.

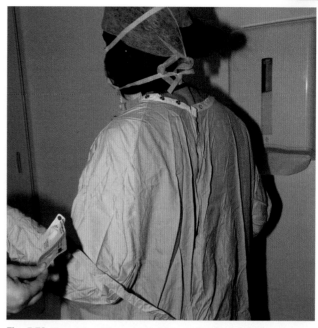

Fig. 5.72 Turn fully whilst your assistant holds the 'dance card'.

Mark Scheme For Examiner

	0	1	2	3
Introduction and General Advice				
Wears clean surgical scrubs, theatre shoes and surgical cap				
Removes rings, watches and jewellery and locks away personal possessions				
Ensures nails are cut short and no nail polish is worn				
Procedure Preparation				
Washes hands, puts on surgical face mask				
Sets up sterile field on the trolley				
Opens surgical gown and correctly sized gloves on trolley				
Obtains hand scrubber packet				
Scrubbing Up				
Cleans fingernails with nail pick and hand scrubber				
Washes hands and arms twice (stops at elbows)				
Washes hands and arms a third time (stops at forearm)				
Allows excess water to drip off arms (does not shake arms), and turns off taps with elbows				
Dries hands using sterile paper towels				
Puts on surgical gown				

Continued

Mark Scheme For Examiner—cont'd

	0	1	2	3
Asks assistant to tie back of gown				
Dons gloves via 'closed' method				
Hands out dance card and ties front of gown				
Finishing				
Walks into theatre with hands in prayer position				
General Points				
Mindful of non-sterile objects in operating theatre				

0= Not attempted
1= Performed, with room for improvement
2= Adequately performed
3= Performed beyond level expected

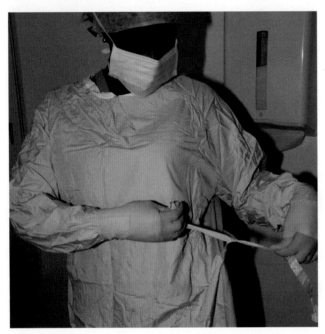

Fig. 5.73 Secure your gown in place by forming a knot.

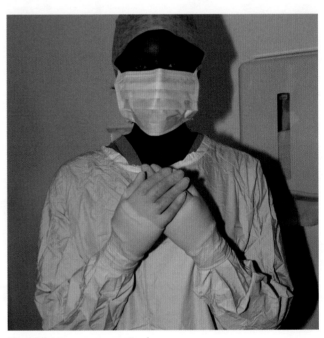

Fig. 5.74 You are now sterile.

❓ QUESTIONS AND ANSWERS FOR CANDIDATE

How long should the first scrub of the day be?
- First scrub should last for 5 min.
- Subsequent scrubs should last for 3 min.

What should you do if you feel unwell or ill whilst scrubbed up?
- Immediately inform the surgeons and theatre staff, walk to the closest wall and sit down with your back against it.

What is the difference between 'sterile' and 'aseptic'?
- 'Aseptic' minimises contamination by *pathogens*.
- 'Sterile' is a complete elimination of *all* microorganisms.

Name the roles of staff likely to be present in an operating theatre.
- Surgeons
- Scrub nurses
- Theatre nurses

- Operating department practitioner
- Anaesthetists
- Theatre support workers
- Radiographers, if required

What is the WHO surgical checklist?

- It is a 19-item checklist that has been developed to reduce errors and adverse events, and increase teamwork and communication in surgery (Fig. 5.75).

 Tip Box

It helps to pinch the nose bridge of the face mask to allow a more comfortable fit. Ensuring that the face mask fits well is of critical importance as it is not sterile and therefore you cannot adjust it once you start to scrub up.

 Fact Box

For operations where there is a high risk of bodily fluids coming into contact with your eyes or face, the hospital should have a stock of face visors and goggles available to you.

GUIDELINES

Maskell, N., British Thoracic Society Pleural Disease Guideline Group, 2010. British Thoracic Society pleural disease guidelines — 2010 update. *Thorax* 65 (8), 667—669. https://doi.org/10.1136/thx.2010.140236.

British Society of Gastroenterology, 2006. Guidelines on the management of ascites. Available at: www.bsg.org.uk/wp-content/uploads/2019/12/BSG-guidelines-on-the-management-of-ascites-in-cirrhosis.pdf. (Accessed 8 June 2022).

WHO guidelines on hand hygiene in health care (No. WHO/IER/PSP/2009/01). World Health Organization; 2009

STATION 6.1: URINALYSIS

SCENARIO

Mrs Manpreet is a 35-year-old female who presents to your clinic with abdominal pain and vomiting. She has been going to the toilet more often than normal, and when she does pass urine, it stings. She is also concerned that her urine is foul smelling. Please ask her to provide a midstream urine sample; perform a urinalysis on it and discuss the result with her.

OBJECTIVES

- Explaining midstream urine samples
- Performing urinalysis
- Interpreting urinalysis findings

GENERAL ADVICE

- Obtain consent.
- Where possible, it is important to obtain a fresh urine sample for analysis.
- When you interpret the urinalysis findings, ensure that you take into consideration the patient's signs and symptoms.
- If you are going to throw the urine sample away after analysis, ensure this is down a sluice and not a domestic sink.

EQUIPMENT CHECKLIST

(Remember to check expiry dates on all equipment [Fig. 6.1]).
- Non-sterile gloves
- Urine reagent strip
- Sterile urine pot
- Paper towel

OBTAINING A MIDSTREAM URINE SAMPLE

1. Give the patient a sterile midstream urine pot – this usually contains boric acid.

2. Ask them to clean their external genitalia with water and tissue.
3. Ask them to pass a small amount of urine into the toilet.
4. Then, without stopping the flow of urine, catch some into the pot to fill to the line.
5. Advise the patient that they can empty their bladder into the toilet.
6. Immediately place the cap on to the urine pot.

PERFORMING A URINE DIPSTICK

1. Give the patient a sterile universal pot and ask them to provide a urine sample.
2. Wash your hands.
3. Put on gloves.
4. Inspect the urine sample – Note whether it looks cloudy, dark yellow or red, or if there are any sediments in it.
5. Remove the cap of the urine container – Note any smell.

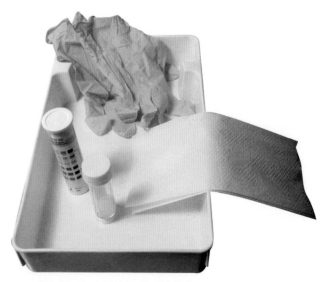

Fig. 6.1 Equipment required to perform urinalysis.

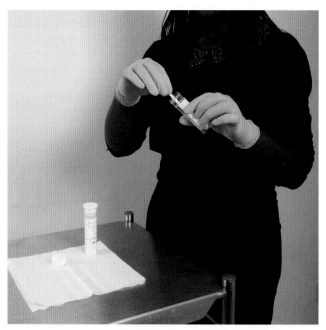

Fig. 6.2 Fully immerse the dipstick.

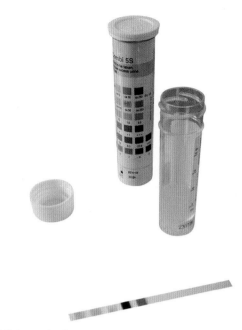

Fig. 6.3 Leave the dipstick horizontal whilst waiting for the chemicals to react.

6. Check the expiry date of the dipstick on the container and remove one dipstick.
7. Place the dipstick in the urine for 2–3 s, ensuring that all the reagents on the dipstick are immersed in the urine (Fig. 6.2).
8. Remove the dipstick.
9. Place the dipstick horizontally onto a flat surface or paper towel to ensure that the chemicals do not mix (Fig. 6.3).
10. Leave the dipstick to dry for the specified time (found on the reagent strip container).
11. Look at each reagent on the dipstick in turn. With each reagent, look at the corresponding colour on the tub (the tub will have a colour code on its side so that you can interpret the results and identify if the value is normal or high [Fig. 6.4]).
12. Document the findings in the patient notes and report back to the patient.

FINISHING

1. Label the pot and accompanying laboratory form with patient details and send to the lab.
2. Remove gloves and wash hands.
3. Discuss your findings with the patient.

DOCUMENT THE PROCEDURE

Document under the following headings:
- Urinalysis performed
- Type of sample: Midstream, catheter, etc.

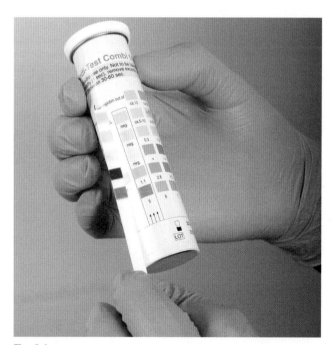

Fig. 6.4 Interpret the results using the chart on the dipstick bottle.

- Date, time and place
- Indications for the procedure
- Patient consent
- Results

INTERPRETATION

All of the results need to be interpreted in the context of the patient. A raised glucose or urinalysis does not necessarily mean that the patient has diabetes. For example, glycosuria can be normal in the context of pregnancy.

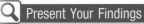
Present Your Findings

Mrs Manpreet is a 35-year-old female who presented with symptoms of a urinary tract infection (UTI). Urinalysis demonstrated nitrites +++, leukocytes +++, blood +; therefore, I have started her on a course of trimethoprim and sent her urine sample for microscopy, culture and sensitivity (MC&S).

APPEARANCE	INFERENCE
Red	Can indicate haematuria
Cloudy	Can indicate infection
Faeculent	Colovesical fistula or contaminated sample
SMELL	
Foul	Infection
Sweet	Diabetic ketoacidosis
Faeculent	Colovesical fistula or contaminated sample
BLOOD	
Positive	Haematuria or haemoglobinuria
False positive	Menstrual blood
KETONES	
Raised	Diabetic ketoacidosis, starvation
NITRITES AND LEUKOCYTES	
Nitrite positive	Suggests bacterial infection
Leukocyte positive	Suggests inflammation and possible infection
PROTEIN	
Raised	Renovascular, glomerular or tubulo-interstitial renal disease
	Pre-eclampsia and hypertension
	Benign due to exercise or postural
	Nephrotic syndrome
GLUCOSE	
Raised	Diabetes
	Pregnancy
	Steroid use
SPECIFIC GRAVITY	
High value	Dehydration
	Heart failure
	Liver failure
	Syndrome of inappropriate antidiuretic hormone (SiADH)
pH	
Alkaline	Can indicate urinary tract infection (UTI) with urea-splitting organisms (e.g. *Proteus*)
Acidic	Can indicate urinary stones made of uric acid and cystine

Mark Scheme for Examiner

	0	1	2	3
Introduction and General Advice				
Introduces self and washes hands				
Confirms patient's identity with three points of identification				
Explains procedure, identifies concerns and obtains consent				
Obtaining Midstream Urine Sample				
Provides patient with sterile specimen pot				
Asks for a midstream urine sample				
Explains how to collect a midstream urine sample				
Urine Dipstick				
Washes hands, dons non-sterile gloves				
Checks expiry date of reagent sticks				
Inspects sample				

Continued

Mark Scheme for Examiner—cont'd

	0	1	2	3
Removes cap and notes odour				
Removes a single dipstick from container				
Dips the urine for 2–3 s				
Places dipstick on flat surface and leaves for specified time				
Uses the colour chart of dipstick container to analyse results				
Finishing				
If indicated, sends sample away; otherwise, disposes of sample				
Removes gloves and washes hands				
Disposes of equipment and cleans work surface				
Interpretation				
Comments on: Blood, ketones, nitrites, leukocytes, protein, glucose, specific gravity and pH				
Discusses the dipstick findings in relation to the patient's symptoms				
Documents findings and management plan in patient's notes				

0 = Not attempted
1 = Performed, with room for improvement
2 = Adequately performed
3 = Performed beyond level expected

❓ QUESTIONS AND ANSWERS FOR CANDIDATE

When might you get a false-positive glucose test on a urine dip?

- The presence of other substances in the urine can interfere with the test strips and give a false positive.
- Examples include: Aspirin, penicillin, isoniazid, vitamin C and cephalosporins.

What does the presence of red-cell casts on light microscopy suggest?

- Glomerulonephritis

Give three causes of haematuria.

- Kidney: Malignancy, calculi, trauma, glomerulonephritis, pyelonephritis, interstitial nephritis, infarction, polycystic kidney disease
- Ureter: Malignancy, calculi, trauma
- Bladder: Malignancy, calculi, trauma, infection
- Urethra and prostate: Malignancy, stone, trauma, benign prostatic hypertrophy
- General: Anticoagulants; for example, warfarin, exercise, paroxysmal nocturnal haematuria
- Not true haematuria: May be vaginal bleeding or menstruation. May not be blood at all (beetroot can give similar appearance, as can certain drugs; for example, rifampicin)

What methods are available for collecting urine samples in a baby?

- Clean-catch urine: Waiting for urine with a sterile pot after the nappy has been removed and the surrounding area has been cleaned (parents should be told to ask for a new sterile pot if it gets contaminated)
- Supra-pubic aspiration (ultrasound-guided)
- Catheter sample

What are urinary Bence Jones proteins?

- A protein that is a section of the antibodies produced by myeloma cells, which the body removes through the urine

 Tip Box

Don't throw away a urine sample after the dipstick is done — wait until a decision is made as to whether it needs to be sent for further investigation.

 Fact Box

Further Urine Investigation

- **A pregnancy test** is important in all fertile women presenting with abdominal pain.
- If there is evidence of a UTI (leukocytes, nitrites, blood, protein), send the urine sample for **MC&S**.
- If there is a concern about myeloma (bone pain, anaemia, renal failure, elevated calcium, proteinuria), send the urine for **protein electrophoresis**.
- **Urine microscopy** can reveal red-cell casts. These occur in the context of glomerulonephritis. In this setting, you need to inform the lab that you are specifically looking for pathological casts on microscopy and the sample will be analysed as soon as practical after being produced, ideally whilst still warm.
- Urine can be tested for **microalbuminuria** in patients who have diabetes mellitus. This is a screening test for nephropathy.
- Protein:creatinine ratios (or urinary PCRs) are useful in quantifying the extent of a patient's proteinuria. A patient has nephrotic-range proteinuria when they are passing more than 3 g/24 h.

STATION 6.2: MALE URETHRAL CATHETERISATION

SCENARIO

Mr Gear has not urinated following an elective operation he had last night and is becoming distressed by abdominal pain. An examination reveals a soft non-tender suprapubic mass which, when palpated deeply, makes Mr Gear feel like he wishes to pass urine. You diagnose acute urinary retention and feel that he requires a urethral catheter. Having already obtained his consent, demonstrate this procedure on the mannequin provided.

OBJECTIVE

• Learn how to perform male catheterisation

GENERAL ADVICE

• Confirm that the patient understands what is going to happen and is happy to continue.
• Obtain consent.
• Always ask for a chaperone.

EQUIPMENT CHECKLIST

(Remember to check expiry dates on all equipment [Fig. 6.5].)
• Procedure trolley
• Sharps bin: Sharps bin should always be taken to the point of care.
• Disposable bag (for rubbish)
• Catheterisation pack (including disposable dish, plastic pots, cotton swabs and sterile drape)
• Two sachets of sterile water or 0.9% saline, according to Trust policy
• Two pairs of sterile gloves
• Local anaesthetic (LA) gel or lubricant, according to Trust policy
• 21-gauge needle
• 10-mL syringe
• Sterile water vial (often pre-drawn up with the catheter)
• Large incontinence pad

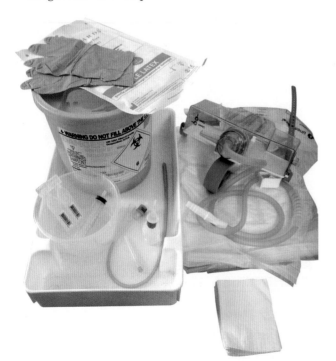

Fig. 6.5 Equipment required to perform male urethral catheterisation.

• Single-use disposable apron
• Male catheter
• Catheter bag (leg bag if appropriate for the patient)
• Sterile universal container (if collecting urine sample)

EXPLAINING CATHETERISATION TO THE PATIENT

1. A urinary catheter is a tube that is placed into the bladder through the hole in the end of your penis, called the urethra, and attached to a bag that collects the urine.
2. You will need to be exposed from your belly button to your knees and lie with your legs slightly apart.
3. Initially, the genitalia will be cleaned and then some anaesthetic gel will be inserted into the urethral meatus to make the procedure more comfortable.
4. The catheter will then be inserted and held in place using a balloon.
5. It is really important that if you feel any pain you tell a nurse or doctor immediately.

CATHETER SELECTION

• **Size:** Use the smallest catheter you can. Normally 14 Ch is used in males and 12 Ch in females.
• **Length:** A male catheter is approximately 40 cm; a female catheter is approximately 25 cm.
• **Material:** Silicone or hydrogel (lasts up to 3 months) or coated latex (lasts up to 4 weeks). Remember to ask about allergies. A patient with latex allergies should have an all-silicone catheter and you should use non-latex gloves.

PERFORMING CATHETERISATION

PREPARE PROCEDURE TROLLEY

1. Clean your hands.
2. Clean the trolley according to local policy.
3. Place a sharps bin on the bottom of your trolley.
4. Open the disposable rubbish bag and attach it to the side of the trolley.
5. Gather your equipment and check the expiry dates.
6. Open the catheterisation pack using a sterile non-touch technique (NTT) on the centre of the trolley.
7. Then open the packaging and drop the lubricant, sachets, gloves and catheter onto the aseptic field.
8. Open the packaging of the catheter bag.
9. If not pre-prepared, draw up sterile water using a 21-gauge needle and a 10-mL syringe. After use, place the needle in the sharps bin.

PREPARE THE PATIENT

1. Expose and position the patient supine but keep him covered with a blanket or towel until just before the procedure, ensuring patient dignity.
2. Put the incontinence pad under the patient.
3. Wash your hands thoroughly, put on a single-use disposable apron and put on sterile gloves.
4. Place a sterile drape with the central hole over the penis (leaving the penis exposed).

ASEPSIS AND ANAESTHESIA

1. Ask the assistant to empty both sterile water sachets into a plastic pot.
2. Soak the cotton swabs in water.
3. Hold the penis with your non-dominant hand and retract the prepuce/foreskin. This hand is now contaminated and should not touch the aseptic trolley.
4. With the right hand, clean the penis in circles beginning at the urethra and moving progressively outwards. Repeat this at least three times.
5. Dispose of the swabs in a disposable rubbish bag.
6. Holding the penis in your non-dominant hand, apply some upwards traction and insert the tip of the lubricant syringe into the urethral meatus (Fig. 6.6).
7. Administer the entire lubricant syringe, allowing some to coat the glans.
8. Leave the lubricant for 5 min to take effect.
9. Remove gloves, wash hands and put on a second pair of sterile gloves.

INSERTING THE CATHETER

1. Place the disposable dish between the patient's legs so that once the catheter is in, urine does not spill onto the bed sheets.
2. Hold the catheter between your thumb and forefinger in your dominant hand.
3. Hold the base of the penis with the non-dominant hand. Apply gentle upward traction to the penis, while inserting the catheter with the other hand into the urethral meatus.
4. Insert the catheter using NTT by touching only the packaging, i.e. insert directly from sterilising packaging (without taking the catheter completely out of the packaging) (Fig. 6.7).
5. Use steady, gentle pressure and never force a catheter.
6. Advance the catheter until urine is seen to flow into the container.
7. Then, once urine is seen to be draining, advance the catheter by another 2.5 cm.
8. If no urine is seen draining, advance the catheter to the fork at the end.
9. Attach the sterile water syringe to the balloon port of the catheter and insert 10 mL slowly (Fig. 6.8). *Stop* if there is pain or high resistance.
10. Attach the catheter to the catheter bag by removing the cap from the tubing and plugging the plastic tube end into the catheter (Fig. 6.9).
11. Replace the prepuce.
12. If there is a leg bag, attach it to the leg. Larger collection bags may be attached to the side of the patient's bed.
13. Clean the patient, remove the incontinence pad and ensure dignity by rearranging bed clothes.

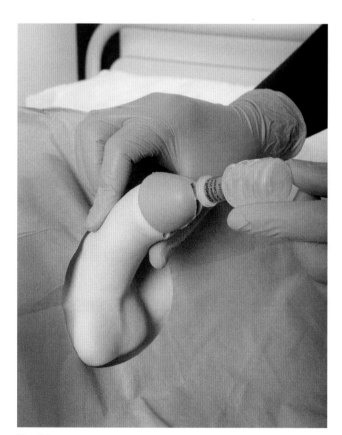

Fig. 6.6 Use anaesthetic gel prior to catheterisation.

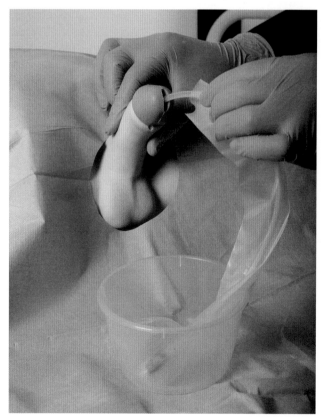

Fig. 6.7 Carefully insert the catheter.

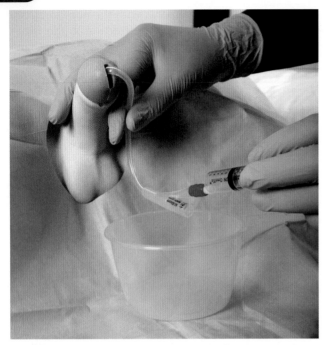

Fig. 6.8 Inflate the balloon using sterile water into the side port.

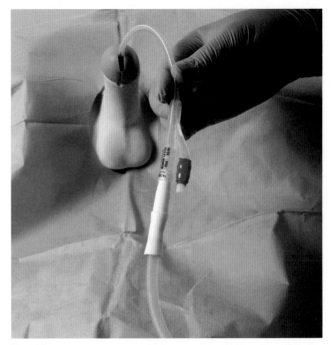

Fig. 6.9 Attach a drainage bag.

14. Dispose of waste.
15. Clean the trolley according to local policy.
16. Remove gloves and decontaminate hands.
17. Tell the patient to report any pain or other concerns to the nursing staff.
18. Document insertion of catheter.

DOCUMENT THE PROCEDURE

You need to document the procedure in the medical notes (often a sticker from the catheter pack is provided for this purpose). Document the procedure, writing the following points:

- Catheterisation performed
- Consent obtained and chaperone present
- Date and time of insertion
- Reason for insertion
- Size, length and material of catheter
- Ease with which catheter passed
- Colour of urine drained
- Volume of sterile water inserted into balloon
- Residual volume of urine (5–10 min after insertion)
- Sign and print your name under your entry

Mark Scheme for Examiner

	0	1	2	3
Introduction and General Advice				
Introduces self and washes hands				
Confirms patient's identity with three points of identification				
Explains procedure, identifies concerns and obtains consent				
Asks for a chaperone				
Positions and exposes the patient				
Chooses the correct size, material and type of catheter				
Procedure Preparation				
Cleans hands				
Obtains equipment and checks expiry dates				
Cleans the trolley				
Prepares trolley and equipment				
If not provided, draws up sterile water into a syringe using a green needle				
Procedure				
Applies single-use apron, washes hands and dons non-sterile gloves				
Places sterile drape, leaving the central hole for the penis				

Continued

Mark Scheme for Examiner—cont'd

	0	1	2	3
Asks assistant to put sterile water into the plastic pot				
Cleans the genitalia, including the urethral opening				
Administers the lubricant correctly				
Removes gloves, washes hands and puts on second pair of sterile gloves				
Places disposable dish between the legs to catch the urine				
Holds the penis in the non-dominant hand and applies upward traction				
Inserts the catheter slowly using NTT until urine passes into the dish or pain/resistance is experienced				
Inflates the balloon with 10 mL sterile water (asks if this is painful and stops if it is)				
Connects catheter to catheter bag				
Replaces the prepuce				
Instructs patient to inform someone if any pain occurs				
Disposes of equipment and cleans tray				
Removes gloves and washes hands				
Documents procedure in the patient's notes				
General Points				
Talks to the patient throughout the procedure				
Uses aseptic technique throughout				
Disposes of sharps and clinical waste appropriately				

0 = Not attempted
1 = Performed, with room for improvement
2 = Adequately performed
3 = Performed beyond level expected

❓ QUESTIONS AND ANSWERS FOR CANDIDATE

When would you think about inserting a urethral catheter?
- To relieve urinary retention
- To monitor urine output in a critically ill patient
- To collect uncontaminated urine for diagnosis

What are the potential risks of urethral catheterisation?
- Infection
- Trauma
- Bladder spasm
- Paraphimosis

How could you damage urethral sphincters during urethral catheterisation?
- If the balloon was inflated in the urethra, this can lead to complete urinary incontinence.

When would you use a three-way catheter?
- Urinary retention
- Urinary output measurement
- After urological surgery
- Clot retention requiring bladder irrigation
- Therapeutic, e.g. clot removal

How would you manage a patient who developed paraphimosis?
- Analgesia
- Reduction of paraphimosis — via manual pressure, application of dextrose-soaked gauze, or the Dundee technique

 Tip Box

Make sure you carefully select the right catheter for your patient, paying particular attention to the length. You must never use a female catheter in a male patient.

 Fact Box

Males have a longer urethra compared to females, and therefore they are treated with a longer course of antibiotics, usually for 7 days.

STATION 6.3: FEMALE URETHRAL CATHETERISATION

SCENARIO

Mrs Shannon is a 75-year-old woman who comes into the emergency department in shock. You have been asked by your registrar to insert a catheter to monitor her fluid balance.

OBJECTIVE

- Learn how to perform female catheterisation

GENERAL ADVICE

The same general principles, equipment, explanation and preparation apply to female catheterisation as stated in station 6.2 on male catheterisation. But remember:

- To place a sterile drape over the patient with the female external genitalia exposed
- Female catchers are shorter and normally smaller than male ones

EQUIPMENT CHECKLIST

(Remember to check expiry dates on all equipment [Fig. 6.10].)

- Procedure trolley
- Sharps bin: Sharps bin should always be taken to the point of care.
- Disposable bag (for rubbish)
- Catheterisation pack (including disposable dish, plastic pots, cotton swabs and sterile drape)
- Two sachets of sterile water or 0.9% saline, according to Trust policy
- Two pairs of sterile gloves
- LA gel or lubricant, according to Trust policy
- 21-gauge needle
- 10-mL syringe
- Sterile water vial (often pre-drawn up with the catheter)
- Large incontinence pad
- Single-use disposable apron
- Female catheter
- Catheter bag (leg bag if appropriate for the patient)
- Sterile universal container (if collecting urine sample)

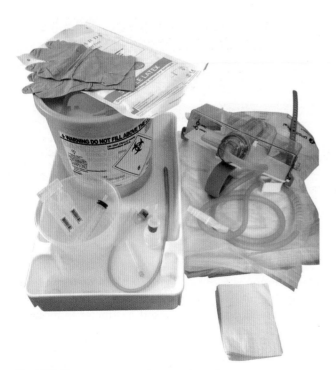

Fig. 6.10 Ensure you prepare your equipment

EXPLAINING CATHETERISATION TO THE PATIENT

1. A urinary catheter is a tube that is placed into the bladder through your urethra and attached to a bag that collects the urine.
2. You will need to be exposed from your belly button to your knees and lie with your legs slightly apart.
3. Initially, the genitalia will be cleaned and then some anaesthetic gel will be inserted into the urethral meatus to make the procedure more comfortable.
4. The catheter will then be inserted and held in place using a balloon.
5. It is really important that if you feel any pain you tell a nurse or doctor immediately.

PERFORMING CATHETERISATION

ASEPSIS AND ANAESTHESIA

1. Ask the assistant to empty both sterile water sachets into a plastic pot.
2. Wash hands, don single-use apron and gloves.
3. Soak the cotton swabs in water.
4. Hold the labia apart with the non-dominant hand. This hand is now contaminated and should not touch the aseptic trolley.
5. With the dominant hand, clean the external genitalia anteriorly to posteriorly. Repeat this at least three times.
6. Dispose of the swabs in a disposable rubbish bag.
7. Insert the tip of the lubricant syringe into the urethral meatus.
8. Administer at least 6 mL of lubricant.
9. Leave the lubricant for 5 min to take effect.
10. Remove gloves, wash hands and put on a second pair of sterile gloves.

INSERTING THE CATHETER

1. Place the disposable dish between the patient's legs so that once the catheter is in, urine does not spill onto the bed sheets.
2. Hold the catheter between your thumb and forefinger in your dominant hand.
3. Insert the catheter using NTT by touching only the packaging, i.e. insert directly from sterile packaging (without taking the catheter completely out of the packaging).
4. Use steady gentle pressure and never force a catheter.
5. Advance the catheter until urine is seen to flow into the container.
6. Then, once urine is seen to be draining, advance the catheter by another 2.5 cm.
7. If no urine is seen draining, advance the catheter to the fork at the end.
8. Attach the sterile water syringe to the balloon port of the catheter and insert 10 mL slowly. *Stop* if there is pain or high resistance.

9. Attach the catheter to the catheter bag by removing the cap from the tubing and plugging the plastic tube end into the catheter (Fig. 6.11).
10. If there is a leg bag, attach it to the leg. Larger collection bags may be attached to the side of the patient's bed.
11. Clean the patient, remove the incontinence pad and ensure dignity.

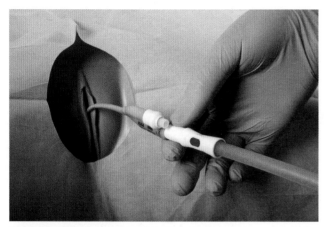

Fig. 6.11 Female catheter in situ.

12. Dispose of waste.
13. Clean the trolley according to local policy.
14. Remove gloves and decontaminate hands.
15. Tell the patient to report any pain or other concerns to the nursing staff.
16. Document insertion of catheter.

DOCUMENT THE PROCEDURE

You need to document the procedure in the medical notes (often a sticker from the catheter pack is provided for this purpose). Document the procedure, writing the following points:

- Catheterisation performed
- Consent obtained and chaperone present
- Date and time of insertion
- Reason for insertion
- Size, length and material of catheter
- Ease with which catheter passed
- Colour of urine drained
- Volume of sterile water inserted into balloon
- Residual volume of urine (5–10 min after insertion)
- Sign and print your name under your entry

Mark Scheme for Examiner

	0	1	2	3
Introduction and General Advice				
Introduces self and washes hands				
Confirms patient's identity with three points of identification				
Explains procedure, identifies concerns and obtains consent				
Asks for a chaperone				
Positions and exposes the patient				
Chooses the correct size, material and type of catheter				
Procedure Preparation				
Cleans hands				
Obtains equipment and checks expiry dates				
Cleans the trolley				
Prepares trolley and equipment				
If not provided, draws up sterile water into a syringe using a green needle				
Procedure				
Applies single-use apron, washes hands and dons non-sterile gloves				
Places sterile drape, leaving the central hole for the external genitalia				
Asks assistant to put sterile water into the plastic pot				
Cleans the genitalia, including the urethral opening				
Administers the lubricant correctly				
Removes gloves, washes hands and puts on a second pair of sterile gloves				
Places a disposable dish between the legs to catch the urine				
Inserts the catheter slowly using NTT until urine passes into the dish or pain/resistance is experienced				
Inflates the balloon with 10 mL sterile water (asks if this is painful and stops if it is)				
Connects catheter to catheter bag				

Continued

Mark Scheme for Examiner—cont'd

	0	1	2	3
Washes hands				
Instructs patient to inform someone if any pain occurs				
Disposes of equipment and cleans tray				
Removes gloves and washes hands				
Documents procedure in the patient's notes				
General Points				
Talks to the patient throughout the procedure				
Uses aseptic technique throughout				
Disposes of sharps and clinical waste appropriately				

0 = Not attempted
1 = Performed, with room for improvement
2 = Adequately performed
3 = Performed beyond level expected

? QUESTIONS AND ANSWERS FOR CANDIDATE

How would you deal with a blocked catheter?
- Attempt to flush the catheter to dislodge any blockages
- A three-way catheter may be needed if there are clots or debris present so regular flushing can occur

What are some long-term complications of catheter use?
- Chronic pyelonephritis
- Nephrolithiasis
- Cystolithiasis
- Chronic renal failure

What are some contraindications to urethral catheterisation (male and female)?
- Patient refusal
- Known urethral strictures
- Enlarged prostate
- Abnormal penile anatomy
- Pelvic or genital trauma

What should normal urine output be?
- 0.5–1.0 mL/kg/h

How would you reduce the risk of catheter-associated UTI?
- Adequate training and education of healthcare professionals and patient on the maintenance of catheters
- Insert catheters only for appropriate indications, and keep the catheter in for the shortest amount of time possible
- Avoid use of urinary catheters for management of incontinence
- Take appropriate infection control measures during catheterisation

 Tip Box

If you are unsure how many millilitres to use to inflate the balloon, then have a look on the catheter packet as there will always be specific instructions. Some varieties of catheter do require more than the standard 10 mL. If you have any doubt, always check.

 Fact Box

Be careful with the antibiotic used to treat UTI in a pregnant female — nitrofurantoin should be avoided if the fetus is at term, whilst trimethoprim should be avoided during the first trimester.

STATION 6.4: SUPRAPUBIC CATHETERISATION

SCENARIO

Mr Sion is a 74-year-old man who presents to hospital with acute urinary retention. He has known urethral strictures and is also under active monitoring for prostate cancer. Attempts have been made to pass a urethral catheter; however these have been unsuccessful. Please perform a suprapubic catheterisation.

OBJECTIVE

- To understand the steps involved in performing suprapubic catheterisation

GENERAL ADVICE

- The safest technique to perform suprapubic catheterisation is to use a flexible cystoscope to visualise the bladder directly. This is usually performed by the urologist under general anaesthetic or LA. Otherwise ultrasound should be used.

- The procedure described below involves suprapubic catheter insertion without the use of cystoscopy and it is therefore vital that the patient's bladder is full.
- There are several different types of suprapubic catheter kits. Although the procedure for insertion is similar for each one, you should always refer to the manual for specific instructions.

EQUIPMENT CHECKLIST

(Remember to check expiry dates on all equipment.)
- Procedure trolley
- Suprapubic catheter kit (including suture disc and prefilled saline syringe to inflate the balloon)
- Two pairs of sterile gloves
- Disposable plastic apron
- Four sterile swabs
- Antiseptic solution and sterile pot
- Two 10-mL syringes (for LA and aspiration)
- 25-gauge needle
- Two 21-gauge needles
- Sterile pack with sterile towels and drape
- 10 mL lidocaine 1%
- Sterile universal container (if collecting urine sample)
- Catheter bag
- Suture kit
- Fine non-absorbable suture
- Clinical waste bag
- Sharps bin: Sharps bin should always be taken to the point of care.

EXPLAINING A SUPRAPUBIC CATHETER TO THE PATIENT

1. A suprapubic catheter is a urinary catheter that is inserted through the abdominal wall, down into the bladder.
2. To perform this procedure, the bladder must be very full.
3. Local anaesthetic is injected around the area of skin where the needle is inserted to numb the skin and provide some pain relief.
4. The catheter is then placed by inserting a needle through the skin, through the abdominal wall and into the bladder.
5. The needle allows the catheter to enter the bladder. Once the catheter is in place the needle is removed.
6. The catheter should then drain freely into a catheter bag.
7. Although it is unlikely, the doctor may be unable to complete the procedure. This means the doctor may need to insert a camera into the bladder to help.

PERFORMING A SUPRAPUBIC CATHETERISATION

PREPARATION

1. Introduce yourself to the patient and obtain written consent.
2. Check the patient's clotting and platelet count.
3. Obtain the equipment.
4. Open the outer packaging of the catheter bag.
5. Expose the patient from nipples to knees and position the patient supine on the bed.
6. Palpate and percuss for the bladder to locate the catheter insertion point and mark 2–3 cm above the pubic symphysis in the midline and well below the superior edge of the palpable bladder. If the bladder cannot be percussed, you must stop the procedure.
7. Open the sterile catheterisation pack and arrange all equipment in the sterile field on your trolley using an aseptic technique.
8. Attach the clinical waste bag to the side of your trolley.
9. Pour the antiseptic solution into the sterile pot and soak the sterile swabs.
10. Wash hands, don apron and the two pairs of sterile gloves provided in the catheter pack.
11. Place the sterile drape around the patient.

ASEPSIS AND ANAESTHESIA

1. Clean the insertion point area in a spiral pattern three times using the swabs soaked in antiseptic solution.
2. Assemble the suprapubic catheter ensuring you check the instructions in the pack.
3. Attach the 21-gauge needle to the 10-mL syringe and aspirate 10 mL of lidocaine 1%.
4. Swap the 21-gauge needle with the 25-gauge needle and infiltrate the LA around the point of insertion, and then use the second 21-gauge needle to infiltrate more deeply.
5. Dispose of sharps appropriately.
6. Remove the outer pair of sterile gloves.

INSERTING THE CATHETER

1. Hold the catheter and puncture needle like a pencil between your thumb and forefinger around 8–10 cm from the distal end.
2. With firm pressure, insert the puncture needle and catheter into the abdomen at the intended puncture site until resistance disappears.
3. Ensure the correct position of the catheter by removing the plug and aspirating urine using a new 10-mL syringe.
4. Remove the puncture needle from the catheter whilst advancing the catheter into the bladder.
5. Inflate the balloon with 10 mL of sterile water from a prefilled syringe (Fig. 6.12).

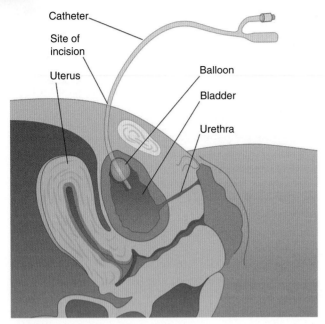

Fig. 6.12 Suprapubic catheter in situ.

6. Dispose of the needle in a sharps bin.
7. Ensure the catheter suture disc is flush with the patient's abdominal wall.
8. Carefully suture the catheter to the abdominal wall using interrupted sutures.

FINISHING

1. Attach the end of the catheter to a universal catheter bag.
2. Ensure the catheter is draining and any clamps are removed.
3. Clean the patient and remove the drape.
4. Clean the trolley and dispose of equipment.
5. Remove gloves and wash hands.
6. Advise the patient to inform a member of staff if they experience any pain or discomfort.

DOCUMENTING THE PROCEDURE

Document under the following headings:
- Suprapubic catheter inserted
- Indications for the procedure
- Patient consent
- Relevant laboratory investigations (e.g. clotting, platelet count)
- Procedure technique, sterile preparation, anaesthetic and amount used, amount of urine drained
- Complications
- Further management required

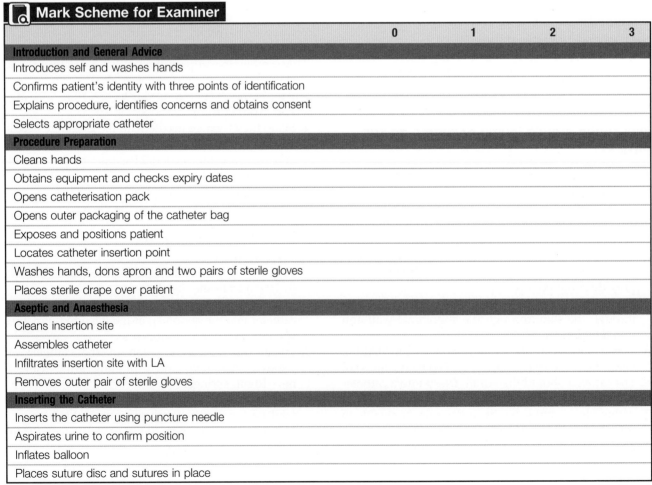

Mark Scheme for Examiner

	0	1	2	3
Introduction and General Advice				
Introduces self and washes hands				
Confirms patient's identity with three points of identification				
Explains procedure, identifies concerns and obtains consent				
Selects appropriate catheter				
Procedure Preparation				
Cleans hands				
Obtains equipment and checks expiry dates				
Opens catheterisation pack				
Opens outer packaging of the catheter bag				
Exposes and positions patient				
Locates catheter insertion point				
Washes hands, dons apron and two pairs of sterile gloves				
Places sterile drape over patient				
Aseptic and Anaesthesia				
Cleans insertion site				
Assembles catheter				
Infiltrates insertion site with LA				
Removes outer pair of sterile gloves				
Inserting the Catheter				
Inserts the catheter using puncture needle				
Aspirates urine to confirm position				
Inflates balloon				
Places suture disc and sutures in place				

Continued

Mark Scheme for Examiner—cont'd

	0	1	2	3
Finishing				
Connects catheter to catheter bag				
Cleans patient				
Instructs patient to inform someone if any pain occurs				
Disposes of sharps and clinical waste appropriately				
Disposes of equipment and cleans tray				
Removes gloves and washes hands				
Documents procedure in the patient's notes				
General Points				
Talks to the patient throughout the procedure				
Aseptic technique throughout				

0 = Not attempted
1 = Performed, with room for improvement
2 = Adequately performed
3 = Performed beyond level expected

? QUESTIONS AND ANSWERS FOR CANDIDATE

What are the contraindications for a suprapubic catheter?

- Severe obesity
- Cognitive impairment
- Clotting disorders
- Undiagnosed haematuria
- Known bladder carcinoma
- Ascites

How often does a suprapubic catheter need changing?
- Every 4–12 weeks

Does a patient require antibiotic prophylaxis for insertion or removal of a urinary catheter?
- Routinely, no
- The following patients may require antibiotic prophylaxis:
  - Mechanical catheter problems, e.g. blockages
  - Infection-related catheter problems, e.g. urethral discharge
  - History of symptomatic UTI after catheter change
  - Experience of trauma associated with insertion or removal of urinary catheter

Name two appropriate antibiotic choices for UTIs.
- Nitrofurantoin
- Cephalosporins, e.g. ceftriaxone and cefotaxime
- Gentamicin

What are the most common microorganisms responsible for urinary tract infections?
- *Escherichia coli*
- *Klebsiella pneumoniae*
- *Proteus mirabilis*
- *Enterococcus faecalis*
- *Staphylococcus saprophyticus*

Tip Box

There are several measures that you can advise your patient of to ensure good catheter care. Good hydration (2–3 L/day) can prevent urinary infections by encouraging drainage. Good personal hygiene will ensure that the catheter insertion site remains healthy. Baths can encourage skin infections, and scented products can sometimes irritate the skin surrounding the insertion site.

Fact Box

If at approximately 6 h post trial without catheter (TWOC) the patient still has >300 mL post-void residual urine, then TWOC is deemed to have been unsuccessful and recatheterisation is indicated.

STATION 7.1: PEAK FLOW

SCENARIO

Mrs Patel has come to your clinic with her 14-year-old son, Sandeep. He has recently been diagnosed with asthma and has been advised to keep a peak flow diary. Please teach him how to perform a peak flow.

GENERAL ADVICE

- Ensure that you have introduced yourself, identified the patient and washed your hands.
- Ensure that your patient has given verbal consent for the procedure and is happy for family/friends present to remain.
- Always make sure there are spare mouthpieces available for the next patient.
- When the patient is given a peak flow monitor they will have their own mouthpiece that they can reuse and wash.

EQUIPMENT CHECKLIST

- Peak flow monitor
- Disposable mouthpiece

EXPLAINING THE PROCEDURE TO THE PATIENT

- People who have been diagnosed with asthma have difficulties with breathing.
- A peak flow monitor can demonstrate how well controlled asthma is over a particular period of time by showing how much air can be exhaled out of the lungs quickly.
- The technique of how to use the peak flow monitor will be demonstrated before you are asked to use it.

OBTAINING A PEAK FLOW READING

After demonstrating peak flow to the patient, ask them to perform the procedure without instruction to check

understanding and technique. Language used may need to be adjusted depending on the child's level of understanding.

1. Ask the patient to stand up or sit up straight.
2. Ensure that the dial on the peak flow monitor is at zero (Fig. 7.1).
3. Make sure that the patient knows not to let his fingers touch the scale or markers during use (Fig. 7.2).
4. Ask the patient to fit the mouthpiece onto the monitor, making sure there is a tight seal around the mouthpiece.
5. Ask the patient to inhale deeply.
6. Ask the patient to place his lips firmly around the mouthpiece.
7. Advise the patient to lift his chin and straighten his back to open the airways fully.

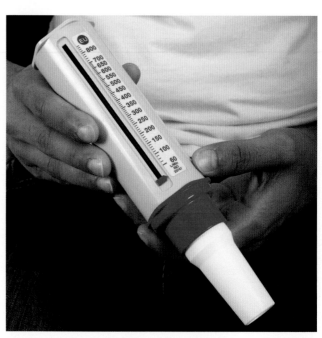

Fig. 7.1 Prepare the peak flow monitor before use.

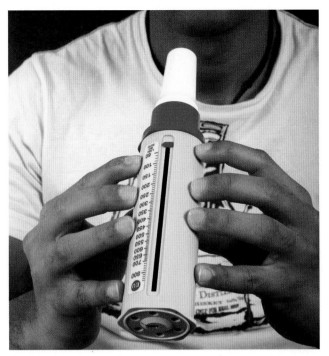

Fig. 7.2 Hold the peak flow meter correctly.

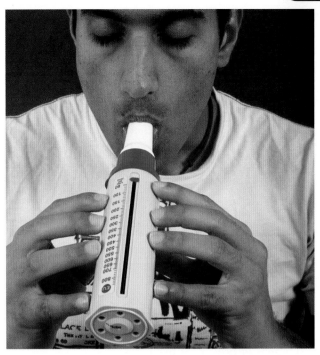

Fig. 7.3 Ask the patient to blow out as hard and as fast as he can.

8. Advise the patient to blow out as hard and as fast as he can. You can use phrases such as 'like you are blowing out the candles on a cake' (Fig. 7.3).
9. Check the dial and record the reading (Fig. 7.4).
10. Move the dial back to zero.
11. Allow the patient a period of rest and then repeat the procedure. **It should be performed three times, and the highest value is the one taken as the peak flow reading at that time.**
12. Compare the reading to a standard chart.
13. Record the results in a peak flow diary, and explain to the patient how to use it.

Mark Scheme for Examiner

	0	1	2	3
Introduction and General Advice				
Introduces self and washes hands				
Confirms patient's identity with three points of identification				
Explains procedure, identifies concerns and obtains consent				
Checks identity of others in the room, and confirms that the patient is happy for them to stay				
Explaining the Peak Flow				
Describes the technique of using the peak flow monitor				
Mentions it should be done three times				
Watches the patient do it without instruction				
Discusses the use of a peak flow diary				
Finishing				
Elicits patient concerns and questions				
Arranges a follow-up appointment if necessary or offers contact details				
Thanks the patient and closes the consultation				
General Points				
Checks patient understanding throughout the consultation, avoiding medical jargon, and offers information leaflet				
Maintains good eye contact, remains polite and engaged with the patient				

0 = Not attempted
1 = Performed, with room for improvement
2 = Adequately performed
3 = Performed beyond level expected

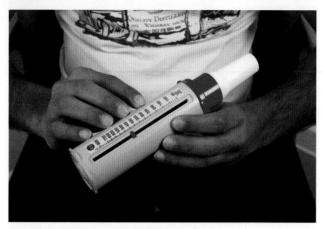

Fig. 7.4 Check the reading for the patient.

QUESTIONS AND ANSWERS FOR CANDIDATE

What factors affect the peak flow result?
- Quality of peak flow technique
- Degree of lung disease
- Height, age and gender

Why is a peak flow diary useful?
- To establish if there is diurnal variation in peak flow associated with asthma
- To establish if there are any environmental triggers associated with asthma

What are the typical changes in lung spirometry in asthma?
- If there is an obstructive defect:
  - The forced expiratory volume in 1 s (FEV_1) is reduced
  - The FEV_1/forced vital capacity (FVC) is reduced
  - >15% improvement in FEV_1 following a β_2 agonist or steroid trial, demonstrating reversibility of airway constriction

Which medications must be used with caution in patients with asthma?
- Non-steroidal anti-inflammatory drugs
- Beta (β)-blockers

In what age group can peak flow be used?
- Starting from 4–5 years old

> **Tip Box**
>
> Advise patients to check their peak flows at least once in the morning and once in the evening so that diurnal variation can be spotted. It is also important to do it at the same times every day.

> **Fact Box**
>
> Best or predicted peak expiratory flow rate is estimated using equations that take into account age and height.

STATION 7.2: INHALER TECHNIQUE

SCENARIO

Mrs Page has come to your clinic with her 7-year-old son, Toby. He has recently been diagnosed with asthma and has been given inhalers. Please teach him how to use an inhaler and a spacer.

OBJECTIVES

- Learning inhaler technique
- Learning how to use a spacer device

GENERAL ADVICE

- It is important that the patient understands the indication for their inhaler, as this would promote better compliance and therefore better disease control.
- Always check the technique before altering medication dosage as poor inhalation technique is common secondary to lack of understanding; this would reduce the amount of drug delivered to the lungs.

EQUIPMENT CHECKLIST

(Remember to check expiry dates on all equipment (Fig. 7.5).)
- Inhaler
- Peak flow meter
- Spacer, if required

EXPLAINING INHALERS TO A PATIENT

- People who have been diagnosed with asthma use inhalers to help with their breathing. Some inhalers are used every day, and some are just used when the patient gets wheezy or thinks they will get wheezy.
- The different colours of the inhalers show that they do different things (Fig. 7.5):
  - The **blue** inhaler is a reliever and should be used when the patient is wheezy as he will feel an immediate improvement in his breathing. If he uses

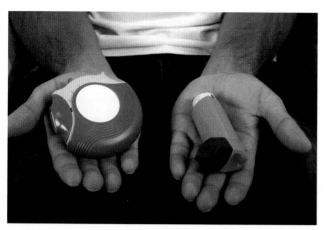

Fig. 7.5 Inhalers come in all shapes and sizes.

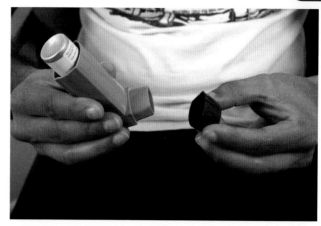

Fig. 7.6 Prepare the inhaler for use.

this more than three times a week, he needs to see his primary care practitioner.

- The **brown/orange** inhaler is a preventer and should be used regularly. He will not notice a difference quickly with this inhaler, but it helps in the long term.
- Other colours may mean that the inhaler contains two different types of medication, e.g. a purple inhaler.

INHALER TECHNIQUE

After demonstrating the inhaler technique to the patient, ask him to perform the procedure without instruction to check understanding and technique. Language used may need to be adjusted depending on the child's level of understanding.

1. Check the expiry date of the inhaler.
2. Ask the patient to stand up or sit up straight, and lift his chin.
3. Shake the inhaler well.
4. Take the cap off the inhaler (Fig. 7.6).
5. Ask the patient to exhale completely.
6. Ask the patient to place his lips firmly around the mouthpiece (Fig. 7.7).
7. Ask the patient to press the canister as he starts to inhale slowly. Remove inhaler from mouth.
8. Ask the patient to hold his breath for 10 s and then breathe out slowly.
9. If more than one puff is required, wait 10 s before repeating the process.

USING A SPACER

It is important to explain the advantages of using a spacer, i.e. even with good inhaler technique, it is hard

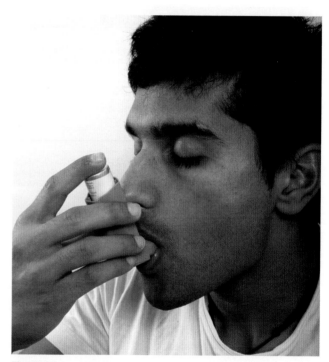

Fig. 7.7 Ensure a tight seal.

to inhale all of the medication, and using a spacer makes this a much easier process as it removes the need to coordinate inhalation and activation.

1. Check the expiry date of the inhaler.
2. Ask the patient to stand up or sit up straight, and lift his chin.
3. Shake the inhaler well.
4. Take the cap off the inhaler.
5. Ask the patient to assemble the spacer and attach the inhaler to it (Fig. 7.8).

6. Ask the patient to exhale completely.
7. Ask the patient to place his lips firmly around the mouthpiece (Fig. 7.9).
8. Ask the patient to press the canister to release a dose into the spacer.
9. Ask the patient to take 5 slow, deep breaths.
10. If more than one puff is required, wait 30 s before repeating the process.
11. Make sure you inform patients about cleaning the spacer. It needs to be washed once a week in warm, soapy water, and left to air dry. Also, spacers need to be replaced every 3 to 6 months.

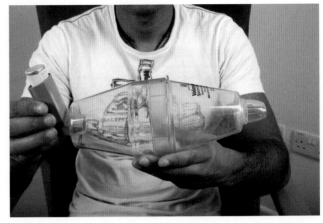

Fig. 7.8 Assemble the equipment correctly.

Mark Scheme for Examiner

	0	1	2	3
Introduction and General Advice				
Introduces self and washes hands				
Confirms patient's identity with three points of identification				
Explains procedure, identifies concerns and obtains consent				
Asks what the patient already knows and if they are on treatment already; asks them to demonstrate technique				
Provides a simple explanation of how a reliever inhaler works				
Inhaler Technique				
Checks expiry date				
Removes cap and shakes inhaler				
Sits upright or stands				
Exhales				
Seals lips around the mouthpiece				
Inhales deeply and presses the canister to release the drug during inhalation				
Removes the inhaler and holds breath for 10 s, then breathes out slowly				
Checks patient understanding				
Asks the patient to demonstrate/repeat				
Using a Spacer				
Explains what a spacer device is and why it is used				
Shakes the inhaler and attaches it to the aerochamber				
Exhales completely. Seals lips around mouthpiece. Presses canister once				
Inhales slowly and deeply; repeats up to 4–5 times				
Provides cleaning advice – rinse and air dry				
Asks the patient to demonstrate/repeat				
Asks the patient if they have any questions				
Finishing				
Arranges a follow-up appointment if necessary or offers contact details				
Thanks the patient and closes the consultation				
General Points				
Checks patient understanding throughout the consultation, avoiding medical jargon, and offers information leaflet				
Maintains good eye contact, remains polite and engaged with the patient				

0 = Not attempted
1 = Performed, with room for improvement
2 = Adequately performed
3 = Performed beyond level expected

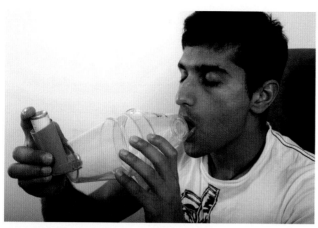

Fig. 7.9 Ensure a tight seal.

❓ QUESTIONS AND ANSWERS FOR CANDIDATE

What are the side effects of inhaled steroids?
- *Candida* infection of the mouth
- Hoarseness
- Rarely:
  - Skin — Easy bruising and thinning
  - Weakened immunity — Instruct patient that they should inform their doctors if they become ill

What are some important questions to ask a patient with chronic asthma?
- What are you like at your worst, and how is your asthma normally?
- Have you ever been admitted to hospital with your asthma? What treatment did you receive?
- Have you ever been admitted to intensive care to help with your breathing?
- Do you use home oxygen, inhalers or nebulisers? Are you on any other medications for asthma?
- How many courses of steroids have you taken in the last year?
- Are there any specific triggers to your asthma?
- Have you had any chest infections in the last year?
- Can you demonstrate your inhaler technique?

Name two different types of inhaler available.
- Metered-dose inhalers
- Breath-activated inhalers — Autohaler, Easi-Breathe
- Dry-powder inhalers — Accuhaler

In the bronchodilator reversibility test, what percentage of improvement in FEV_1 would be regarded as a positive result?
- 12%

Which conditions are included in the atopy triad?
- Atopic eczema or dermatitis
- Asthma
- Allergic rhinitis

 Tip Box

Encourage patients to carry a blue reliever inhaler with them as well as having one at home as it is hard to predict when they will become symptomatic.

 Fact Box

There are different types of spacers. For example:
- Babyhaler: In <2-year-old children (with face mask) — does not have to be upright, listen for five clicks.
- Volumatic: In >2-year-old children (with or without face mak) — should be seated upright.
- Aerochamber with three different-sized masks for infants, children and adults (now the most commonly prescribed spacer in the UK).

STATION 7.3: PREPARING BABY FORMULA MILK

SCENARIO

Mrs. Fenton is a woman with a 2-month-old child. She has decided to stop breastfeeding and wants to use baby formula milk. Please demonstrate to her how to prepare baby formula milk correctly.

OBJECTIVE
- Preparing baby formula milk

GENERAL ADVICE
- It can be difficult to advise on preparing baby formula milk if you have never done it before yourself. Community midwives and health visitors are often in a great position to offer ongoing advice to mothers regarding the care of their newborn, and you can approach them to ask for tips.

EXPLAINING PREPARING BABY FORMULA MILK
- Preparing milk in a sterilised manner is vital. Although rare, bacterial infections in infants can be life-threatening.
- The main method to reduce the risk of bacterial infection is to prepare each feed with boiling water, as this kills any potentially harmful bacteria.
- **It is critical to remember to cool the water fully before giving the feed to the infant.**

PREPARATION
- Ensure you wash your hands with soap and water before handling any of the equipment needed.
- All equipment must be sterilised before each use.
- Clean the work surface before you prepare the formula milk.

PREPARING BABY FORMULA MILK
1. Fill a kettle with fresh cold tap water.
2. Boil the kettle.
3. Leave to cool for 15–30 min (ensuring the temperature of the water is above 70°C).

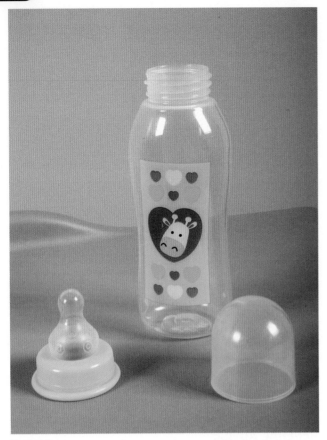

Fig. 7.10 Bottle, teat and cap.

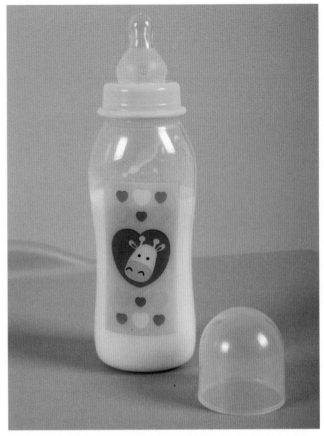

Fig. 7.11 Ensure all of the powder is dissolved before use.

4. Wash your hands with soap and water.
5. Take out the baby's bottle, teat and cap from the steriliser (Fig. 7.10).
6. Stand the baby bottle on the cleaned work surface.
7. Follow the manufacturer's instructions for the formula using the specified amount of formula powder and hot water. Place the water into the bottle first, followed by the powder.
8. Put the teat on to the bottle, holding the edge.
9. Screw the teat onto the bottle.

10. Place the cap over the teat.
11. Shake the bottle firmly until the powder has dissolved.
12. Allow the formula to cool quickly by running the bottle under a cold tap.
13. Test the temperature of the formula using the inside of your wrist. The formula should be at body temperature so should feel tepid to touch, not hot.
14. The formula is now ready to use (Fig. 7.11).

Mark Scheme for Examiner

	0	1	2	3
Introduction and General Advice				
Introduces self and washes hands				
Confirms patient's identity with three points of identification				
Explains procedure, identifies concerns and obtains consent				
Cleans the work surface				
Preparing Baby Formula Milk				
Boils tap water				
Leaves to cool				
Washes hands with soap and water				
Removes equipment from steriliser				
Follows manufacturer's instructions for quantities of water and powder				
Screws teat in place				
Places on cap				
Shakes firmly				
Cools bottle under cold tap water and then tests temperature				

Continued

Mark Scheme for Examiner—cont'd

	0	1	2	3
Finishing				
Ensures workspace is cleaned				
Discusses questions with parents				

0 = Not attempted
1 = Performed, with room for improvement
2 = Adequately performed
3 = Performed beyond level expected

QUESTIONS AND ANSWERS FOR CANDIDATE

Why is it not advisable to give cow's milk to an infant under the age of 1?
- Cow's milk has low levels of some nutrients, specifically iron, vitamin C and vitamin E. Cow's milk can also be a source of bacterial infection as it is not sterile.

How long can prepared baby formula milk be kept unrefrigerated?
- 2 h; thereafter, the formula milk should be discarded

What age would you begin introducing solid foods to babies?
- At 6 months

What are some signs that a baby is ready for solid foods?
- Baby is able to stay in a sitting position and hold their head steady.
- Baby can coordinate their eyes, hands and mouth with the result that food can be placed into the mouth.
- Baby is able to swallow food.

Why would you advise parents against adding sugar and salt to their baby's food?
- Excess sugar could lead to tooth decay.
- Excess salt cannot be processed effectively by immature kidneys.

Tip Box

Always ensure that you use the scoop that is provided with the formula powder to measure the correct amount of powder. If the formula is too concentrated, dehydration can ensue. In contrast, if the formula is too weak, it can eventually lead to faltering growth.

Fact Box

Only prepare feeds at the time they are required. Despite being prepared correctly, formula kept in the fridge is still at risk of becoming infected with bacteria. If absolutely necessary, formula can be kept in the fridge for up to 24 h, but this is not recommended. Any leftover formula should be thrown away or used within 2 h.

Outline

STATION 8.1: HAND WASHING

SCENARIO

Please demonstrate your hand-washing technique.

OBJECTIVES

- To revise the correct method of hand washing
- To understand when the use of soap and water or alcohol gel for hand washing is indicated

GENERAL ADVICE

Each trust will have guidelines adapted from the World Health Organization (WHO) guidelines on the "Five Moments of Hand Hygiene". Ensure that you are familiar with these.

HAND-WASHING PROCEDURE

1. Thoroughly wet hands with warm water.
2. Apply liquid soap or disinfectant from dispenser.
3. Wash hands using the Ayliffe technique (described below):
   - Palm to palm (Fig. 8.1)
   - Palm to palm with fingers interlaced (Fig. 8.2)
   - Back of left-hand fingers against right-hand opposing palms with fingers interlocked, then vice versa (Fig. 8.3)
   - Left thumb clasped in right palm and vice versa (Fig. 8.4)
   - Fingers of right hand clasped in left palm and vice versa (Fig. 8.5)
4. Rinse hands thoroughly.

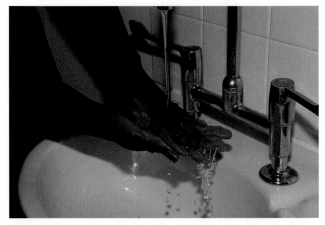

Fig. 8.1 Palm to palm.

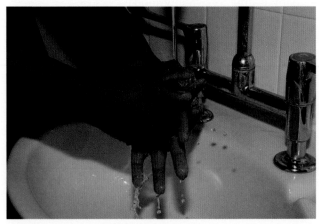

Fig. 8.2 Palm to palm with fingers interlaced.

5. Turn taps off with elbows.
6. Dry hands with paper towel.
7. Dispose of paper towel in clinical waste bin.

Mark Scheme for Examiner

	0	1	2	3
Preparation				
Wets hands with warm water				
Applies soap or disinfectant				
Ayliffe Technique				
Palm to palm				
Fingers intercalated				
Palm over back of hand				
Thumb				
Fingers				
Repeats each action for both hands				
Finishing				
Rinses hands				
Turns off taps with elbows				
Dries hands with paper towel				
Disposes of paper towel				

0 = Not attempted
1 = Performed, with room for improvement
2 = Adequately performed
3 = Performed beyond level expected

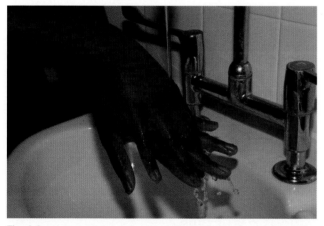

Fig. 8.3 Back of left hand fingers against right hand opposing palms with fingers interlocked, then vice versa.

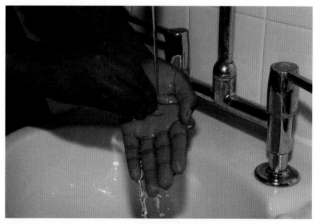

Fig. 8.5 Fingers of right hand clasped in left palm.

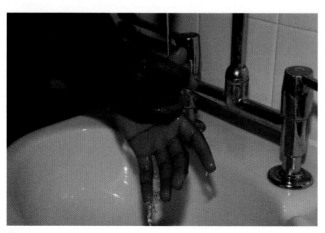

Fig. 8.4 Left thumb clasped in right palm.

? QUESTIONS AND ANSWERS FOR CANDIDATE

What are the "Five Moments of Hand Hygiene"?
- Prior to patient contact
- After patient contact
- Before an aseptic task
- After contact with patient surroundings
- After exposure to bodily fluid

Who must perform hand hygiene?
- Healthcare professionals
- Patients
- Visitors
- Allied health professionals

Can gloves be a substitute for hand washing?
- No; if gloves are to be worn, hands must be washed before the gloves are put on and after they are removed.

How might you prevent hand washing-related dermatitis?

- Regular use of hand moisturisers

What are the four main means of transmission of microorganisms?

- Contact (direct and indirect)
- Respiratory droplets
- Airborne spread
- Common vehicle

 Tip Box

Areas such as the thumbs and tips of the fingers are commonly missed during hand washing. Ensure that you focus on such areas.

 Fact Box

Hands should be washed with soap and water if they are visibly soiled or you have undertaken any procedure that you have used gloves for. Alcohol gel is adequate if hands are not soiled (for example, entering or leaving a hospital ward). Usage of soap and water is also preferable if there is a concern about certain infections, e.g. *Clostridium difficile*.

STATION 8.2: INFECTION CONTROL

SCENARIO

Mrs Tower is a 69-year-old woman who is being cared for on the high-dependency unit. She has been isolated following positive swabs for methicillin-resistant *Staphylococcus aureus* (MRSA), has a long-term urinary catheter and a central venous catheter and is being fed by a nasogastric (NG) tube. Please discuss with the examiner the infection control issues surrounding this patient.

OBJECTIVES

- To understand the infection control aspects of urinary catheters
- To understand the infection control aspects of enteral feeding
- To understand the infection control aspects of central venous catheters

GENERAL ADVICE

- Each Trust will have guidelines for infection control. Ensure that you are familiar with your Trust's policies. Hand washing is discussed in station 8.1, and PPE in Station 8.8.

LONG-TERM URINARY CATHETERS

IMPORTANT INFECTION CONTROL ASPECTS TO CONSIDER WITH REGARD TO URINARY CATHETERS

- Long-term catheters are only used once other methods of management have been considered or tried.
- Catheters should be inserted using an aseptic technique and changed following manufacturer's recommendation.
- Patients with long-term catheters should be educated on managing their catheter using basic infection control principles.
- Patients with a history of recurrent urinary tract infections (UTIs) or cardiac defects should have antibiotic cover when changing catheters.

ENTERAL FEEDING

IMPORTANT INFECTION CONTROL ASPECTS TO CONSIDER WITH REGARD TO ENTERAL FEEDING

- Where possible, enteral feeds should be ready to use. Feeds that require diluting or reconstituting are at higher risk of contamination.
- Enteral feeding tubes should be flushed regularly before and after each use with cooled boiled water or sterile water according to Trust protocol.
- When connecting the feed with the administration system, there should be minimal handling to reduce the infection risk.

CENTRAL VENOUS CATHETERS

IMPORTANT INFECTION CONTROL ASPECTS TO CONSIDER WITH REGARD TO CENTRAL VENOUS CATHETERS

- Central venous catheters must be handled using an aseptic technique, preferably with sterile gloves.
- Dressings over the insertion site should be transparent to allow the site to be assessed for signs of infection, such as erythema, discharge and warmth. Dressings should be changed at least once a week.
- Catheter infection ports are at high risk for infection, so should be cleaned using an alcohol wipe before and after each use.
- Catheter ports should be clearly labelled in accordance with their use. The label is placed at the distal end of the infusion line. The use of each port should be clearly documented in the patient's notes. Examples of possible labels include: blood sampling, medication administration or blood administration.

Mark Scheme for Examiner

	0	1	2	3
Personal Protective Equipment (PPE)				
Discusses indications				
Discusses common PPE, e.g. gloves				
Discusses less common PPE, e.g. respirators				
Long-Term Urinary Catheters				
Discusses catheter insertion				
Discusses antibiotic use				
Discusses basic infection control procedures for long-term catheters				
Enteral Feeding				
Discusses different feeds, e.g. ready-to-use vs those requiring preparation				
Discusses process of giving feeds				
Central Venous Catheters				
Discusses handing central venous catheters				
Discusses monitoring of insertion site				
Discusses labelling catheters				

0 = Not attempted
1 = Performed, with room for improvement
2 = Adequately performed
3 = Performed beyond level expected

❓ QUESTIONS AND ANSWERS FOR CANDIDATE

Which commensals normally colonise our skin?
- *Staphylococcus epidermidis*
- Other coagulase-negative staphylococci, e.g. *Staphylococcus aureus*
- Micrococcus
- Diphtheroids

Name three risk factors for *Clostridium difficile*.
- Over 65 years old
- Multiple or prolonged antibiotic use
- Recent visits/stay in healthcare setting, e.g. care homes or hospitals
- Underlying conditions, e.g. inflammatory bowel disease, kidney disease
- Immunocompromised
- Use of proton pump inhibitors
- Previous abdominal surgery

What are the main antibiotics that are known to increase the risk of *Clostridium difficile* infection?
- Clindamycin
- Co-amoxiclav
- Cephalosporins
- Fluoroquinolones, e.g. ciprofloxacin, levofloxacin

Name three complications *Clostridium difficile* infection.
- Pseudomembranous colitis
- Toxic megacolon
- Perforation of the colon
- Sepsis
- Death

What is the mainstay treatment for *Clostridium difficile* infection?
- If it is the first episode, it is treated with oral vancomycin for 10 days.
- If there have been multiple recurrences, then it is treated with oral vancomycin for 10 days, followed by either a reducing regimen or a pulse regimen.
- Alternatively, it can be treated with metronidazole, usually for 10 to 14 days.

 Tip Box

If you need a refresher in hand hygiene or other infection control-related courses, your place of work should have an infection control lead whom you can approach for this.

 Fact Box

The only indication for oral vancomycin is in the treatment of *Clostridium difficile* infection and enterocolitis infection by certain bacteria; otherwise, the drug is administered intravenously. This is because it is not normally well absorbed and therefore only has a localised effect on infections in the intestines.

STATION 8.3: MANUAL HANDLING

SCENARIO

Mr Counter is an 89-year-old man admitted 3 weeks ago following a stroke. He has reduced power in his left arm and leg and finds it hard to mobilise on the ward. Please discuss how you would assess this patient for a task involving manual handling and describe some of the common manual handling techniques used on the ward.

OBJECTIVES

- To assess a manual handling task for a patient
- To understand independent movement methods
- To understand basic assisted techniques for adults

GENERAL ADVICE

- Each trust will have guidelines for manual handling and hold regular update courses which you should attend. Where possible, patients should be encouraged to mobilise by themselves. If manual handling is required, a full assessment must be made before each task.

MANUAL HANDLING ASSESSMENT

ASSESSMENT OF A MANUAL HANDLING TASK

1. I would need to consider the patient, the nature of the task, the environment and the equipment available.
2. When assessing the patient, I need to consider factors, including their ability, understanding, weight, height and cooperation.
3. When assessing the environment, I need to determine whether it is suitable and safe to undertake the manual handling task, considering lighting, hazards and accessibility.
4. When assessing the equipment available, I need to ensure that I am aware of the equipment within my department, whether it is suitable and safe to use and that the user is trained to use it.

INDEPENDENT MOVEMENT METHODS

DISCUSSION

1. Independent movement methods provide minimal support to patients, allowing them to remain mobile and independent. These methods should only be utilised if they are deemed safe for your patient.
2. These methods involve talking patients through methods to assist with mobilising. Examples of these methods include the following.

Sitting Up From Lying (Fig. 8.6)
Tell the patient:
1. Bend your knees.
2. Roll towards your strong arm.
3. Push up with both arms to sitting.

Shuffling Back Up the Bed (Fig. 8.7)
Tell the patient:
1. Sit upright.
2. Lean forwards.
3. Place both hands behind your hips.
4. Bend both knees.
5. Push down with your hands and lift your buttocks.
6. Push up the bed using your heels, not letting your buttocks drag on the sheets.

Standing from Sitting (Fig. 8.8)
Tell the patient:
1. Shuffle your buttocks to the front of the chair.
2. Place both feet flat on the floor under your knees.
3. Grip the armrest with both hands.
4. Lean forward over your knees.
5. Push upwards using your hands and legs to stand.

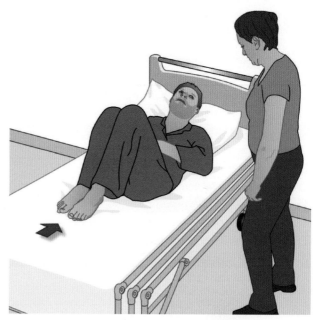
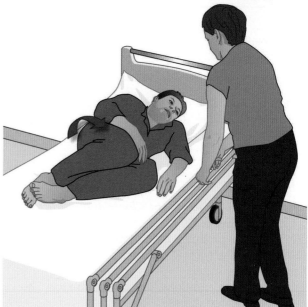
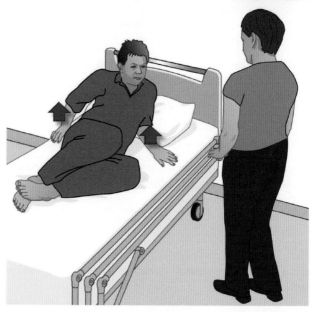

Fig. 8.6 Three steps used to sit from lying.

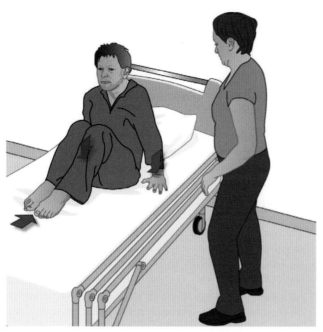

Fig. 8.7 How to direct a patient to shuffle up the bed.

ASSISTED TECHNIQUES

DISCUSSION

1. Assisted techniques are in place to ensure that patients are moved in a safe and careful manner.
2. Where possible, independent movement methods are tried before an assisted technique is used.
3. An assisted technique should only be undertaken following a full manual handling assessment and if the appropriate number of staff to perform the task are available.

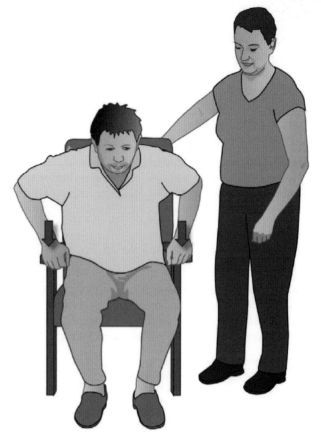

Fig. 8.8 How to stand from sitting.

4. Examples of such techniques include:
   - Turning a patient in bed using a slide sheet
   - Assisting a patient to sit from lying
   - Sliding a patient up the bed using a slide sheet
   - Transferring a patient between beds
   - Assisting a patient to stand from sitting in a chair

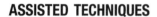

Mark Scheme for Examiner				
	0	1	2	3
Manual Handling Assessment				
Assesses patient — ability, understanding, height, weight, cooperation				
Assesses task				
Assesses environment				
Assesses equipment				
Independent Moving Methods				
Discusses what these methods are				
Discusses some examples				
Discusses which patients they would be indicated in				
Assisted Techniques				
Discusses what these methods are				
Discusses some examples				
Discusses which patients they would be indicated in				

0 = Not attempted
1 = Performed, with room for improvement
2 = Adequately performed
3 = Performed beyond level expected

❓ QUESTIONS AND ANSWERS FOR CANDIDATE

Why does a manual handling assessment have to be undertaken?
- To ensure patient safety
- To ensure staff safety
- To ensure the patient is moved in the best possible way, encouraging independence where possible

Once an assessment has been carried out for a task, does it have to be repeated?
- Only if the patient's ability, understanding or cooperation changes

How would you calculate a patient's body mass index (BMI)?
- BMI is calculated as (weight in kg) divided by (height in m)^2.

What factors are important to take into account when moving and handling a patient?
- The patient's dignity, expectations and wishes
- The patient's ability to communicate

What assistance or equipment might be useful to help a patient's communication?
- Hearing aids
- Visual aids
- Braille equipment if required
- Pen and paper
- Interpreter

 Tip Box

Make sure that you have had adequate training for manual handling and always put your safety first when carrying out specific tasks.

 Fact Box

Each patient who has problems with mobility and needs assistance should have an up-to-date manual handling assessment, usually located in the nursing notes.

STATION 8.4: DEATH CERTIFICATION

SCENARIO

You are asked to verify a death and to write a death certificate. Your patient is Mrs Alice Jayne Morgue, DOB 14.02.1947. She has known angina and passed away today (22.10.2022) in hospital at 22:50. She was admitted 3 days ago with an ST elevated myocardial infarction (STEMI) after collapsing in the street whilst shopping. She was being treated for type 2 diabetes (diagnosed in 1997) and hypertension (diagnosed in 2002). She was not for resuscitation and was found dead in her bed during the night.

OBJECTIVES

- Learning how to verify a death
- Learning how to write a death certificate
- Learning how to complete a cremation form

GENERAL ADVICE

- Remember that the death certificate is an important legal document.
- It enables the death to be formally registered, and only then can the family make arrangements for disposal of the body. Bear in mind as well that, in accordance with certain religious practices, the deceased family member should ideally be buried as soon as possible and therefore the death certificate needs to be filled in as soon as possible.
- The Births and Deaths Registration Act 1953 requires you, as a registered medical practitioner, to certify the cause of death to the best of your knowledge and belief.
- You must identify the underlying cause of death, which must be a specific disease rather than a mechanism of death.
- The death certificate also provides epidemiological information from which mortality data are derived.

DEATH VERIFICATION

Examine the patient to determine the following:
- No response to a painful stimulus (sternal rub or supraorbital pressure)
- Absence of carotid pulse for over 1 min
- Absence of breath sounds of over 1 min
- Absence of heart sounds of over 1 min
- Pupils dilated and unresponsive to light

Always remember to:
- Record the date and time of death in the notes. The time of death is taken when the death is verified and not before
- Leave the patient (mannequin) in a dignified manner, and cover the body with a sheet up to the neck

WRITING A DEATH CERTIFICATE

- Make sure you understand and know the case. You do not have to have been present at the death or have been the doctor who verified it but you must have seen the patient within the last 2 weeks before death.

- Ask about the specific hospital protocol for death certificates. Some hospitals expect you, as a junior doctor, to discuss the death with a consultant before issuing the certificate.
- Write in block capitals and in black ink.
- Avoid medical abbreviations.
- Write the patient's full name.
- When writing the date of death, put the date in words.
- State the place of death.
- Remember to check the patient's employment history, as some industrial diseases attract financial compensation (e.g. exposure to asbestos).

You must circle one of the following:
- The certified cause of death takes account of information obtained from postmortem.
- Information from postmortem may be available later.
- Postmortem is not being held.

You must circle one of the following:
- Seen after death by me
- Seen after death by another medical practitioner but not by me
- Not seen by a medical practitioner

 Tip Box

As a junior doctor you may be the one who fills out death certificates and cremation forms. It is important that you make sure you don't rush these forms and you discuss the cause of death with the team to confirm that the details you write down are correct. If in any doubt regarding what to put on the form, then the local coroner's officers are a good resource and may be able to help.

CAUSE OF DEATH

- Write the cause (e.g. myocardial infarction) rather than mode of death (coma, syncope and cardiac arrests are modes of death).
- If you do not know the cause of death, you may not be able to issue the death certificate.
- State whether the case has been reported to the coroner (or Procurator Fiscal in Scotland).

PART I

- State the disease or condition directly leading to death on the first line, Part Ia.
- Complete the sequence of conditions leading to death on subsequent lines.

For example, Part Ia: Intrapulmonary haemorrhage; Part Ib: Squamous cell carcinoma of the lung.

PART II

- State significant conditions or diseases that contributed to the death, but that are not part of any sequence leading directly to death; for example, diabetes mellitus.
- The duration of all conditions listed in Parts I and II should be listed.
- Print your name clearly after your signature, and add your medical qualification as registered with the General Medical Council. If your medical qualification was obtained in another country, state which university town it was obtained in and the year it was awarded.
- Give the name of the consultant responsible for the care of the patient.

Copy what has been written on the death certificate into the medical notes, and in the death certificate booklet on the stub in the spaces provided. It is often useful to note which family members were present at the time of death and whether the primary care clinician has been informed yet.

CREMATION FORMS

- Do not complete the cremation form until you know that the case is not being investigated by the coroner or procurator fiscal and a death certificate has been issued.
- The patient must have been seen by the certifying doctor in the last 2 weeks of life.
- The first part can be filled in by any doctor, but that doctor must have seen the patient alive within the last 2 weeks of life and then seen and examined the body after dearth.
- The presence of pacemakers or any type of radioactive implant must be recorded as these may preclude cremation unless they are removed.
- All parts of the form must be completed in full and then signed.
- After filling out the first part of the form, a second doctor (who has been fully registered for more than 5 years) must fill out the second part.
- The form should not be given to the relatives but will be passed to the undertakers, usually via the mortuary staff or bereavement officers.

Please complete the death certificate for Mrs Morgue.

Medical certificate of cause of death

Name of deceased

Date of death	Day	Month	Year		Time of death	Hour	Min

Place of death

Cause of death

I hereby certify that to the best of my knowledge and belief, the cause of death was as stated below:

Approximate interval between onset and death
Years Months Days

1. Disease or condition directly leading to death

a.) _____

Antecedent causes

Morbid conditions, if any, giving rise to above cause, stating the underlying condition last

b.) _____

c.) _____

d.) _____

2. Other significant conditions contributing to the death, but not related to the disease or condition causing it

_____

_____

Please tick the relevant box

Post mortem

PM1 ☐ Post mortem has been done and information is included above

PM2 ☐ Post mortem information may be available later

PM3 ☐ No post mortem is being done

Procurator fiscal/coroner

PF ☐ This death has been reported to the procurator fiscal/coroner

Extra information for statistical purposes

X ☐ I may later be able to supply the Registrar General with additional information

Attendance on deceased

A1 ☐ I was in attendance upon the deceased during last illness

A2 ☐ I was not in attendance upon the deceased during last illness: the doctor who was is unable to provide the certificate

A3 ☐ No doctor was in attendance on the deceased

Signature _____

Name in BLOCK CAPITALS _____

Official address _____

Date: _____

For a death in hospital

Name of the consultant responsible _____

- -

Counterfoil – Medical certificate of cause of death

Name of deceased _____

Date of death _____

Place of death _____

Please circle as appropriate			
Post mortem	PM1 or	PM2 or	PM3
Procurator fiscal/coroner	PF		
Extra information	X		
Attendance on deceased	A1	A2	A3

Cause of death

I (a) _____

(b) _____

(c) _____

(d) _____

II _____

Date of certificate _____

Mark Scheme for Examiner

	0	1	2	3
Introduction and General Preparation				
Introduces self to relatives, if present				
Washes hands				
Explains the process of death verification				
Verification of Death				
Assesses for a painful stimulus				
Palpates for a carotid pulse for 1 min				
Auscultates for heart sounds and breath sounds for 1 min each				
Assesses pupil size and response				
Documents the death in the notes correctly				
Leaves the patient in an appropriate state				
Writing a Death Certificate				
Writes in black ink, block capitals, without abbreviations				
Fills in the patient's details, place, date and time of death correctly				
Chooses appropriate option about postmortem, reporting to procurator fiscal/coroner and notes if the doctor filling out the certificate was present at time of death				
Fills in cause of death appropriately				
Fills in comorbidities appropriately				
Fills in personal details and consultant details				
Signs the document				

0 = Not attempted
1 = Performed, with room for improvement
2 = Adequately performed
3 = Performed beyond level expected

❓ QUESTIONS AND ANSWERS FOR CANDIDATE

Name five examples when a death might be reported to a coroner (or procurator fiscal).

- Any uncertified death, i.e. for which the clinician is unable or unwilling to issue a death certificate
- Any death that is sudden and unexpected, or that is due to any violent, suspicious or unexplained cause
- Any death for which the cause is known but the patient has not been seen within the last 2 weeks of life
- Any death resulting from an accident at work or arising out of the use of a vehicle, or involving burns or scalds, or a fire or an explosion, or any other similar cause. This includes deaths occurring as a late result of trauma, i.e. months afterwards
- Any death due to poisoning, including drug overdose (even as a late result)
- Any death resulting from an industrial disease
- Any death in hospital occurring within 24 h of admission
- Any death where circumstances indicate that suicide is a possibility
- Any death where there are indications that it occurred as a result of medical mishap
- Any death following an abortion or attempted abortion

- Any death where the circumstances seem to indicate fault or neglect on the part of another person or organisation, including hospitals
- Any death occurring as a result of food poisoning or a notifiable infectious disease
- Any death of a foster child

Whom can you consult if you need help filling out the death certificate?
- Senior colleagues
- Coroner

What is the difference between decorticate and decerebrate movements?
- Decorticate posturing is abnormal flexion of the upper limbs with extension of the lower limbs. It involves slow flexion of the elbow, wrist and fingers with adduction and internal rotation at the shoulder.
- Decerebrate posturing is adduction and internal rotation of shoulder, extension at the elbows with pronation of the forearm and flexion of the fingers.

Which professionals in the hospital are available for emotional and spiritual support to patients, relatives and hospital staff?
- Hospital chaplain — they can provide support during a crisis as well as during ongoing recovery and through bereavements

What are the three different types of death certificate?
- Medical certificate of cause of death (form 66)
- Neonatal death certificate (form 65)
- Certificate of stillbirth (form 34)

 Tip Box

The relatives may wish to remain while you verify the death of the patient. If this is the case, make sure you explain what you are going to do as otherwise they may be distressed when you are assessing for a response to a painful stimulus.

 Fact Box

It is important to bear in mind religious practices when it comes to deaths and funerals. For example, many muslims prefer to bury their loved ones as soon as possible; therefore, it is important that the death certificates can be issued as soon as possible as well.

STATION 8.5: PERSONAL PROTECTIVE EQUIPMENT (PPE)

SCENARIO

Mr Gerald is a 59-year-old man who has presented with a persistent cough and pyrexia at 38°C. His chest X-ray shows bilateral patchy consolidation and is currently being treated as COVID-19 pneumonia. Please discuss with the examiner the use of PPE in such circumstances, and explain to the examiner what you know about other forms of PPE.

OBJECTIVES

- To understand the infection control aspects of PPE
- To be able to list the appropriate PPE that should be used when performing clinical procedures

GENERAL ADVICE

- Each Trust will have guidelines for infection control. Ensure that you are familiar with your Trust's policies. This station is specific to the use of PPE; other infection control and hand washing are discussed in the previous stations.

EXPLAINING PPE

- PPE reduces infection passing between me and my patient. It describes items such as gloves, aprons, face masks and eye protection which are used during certain procedures to prevent microorganisms from coming into contact with you or your clothing.

- I have seen gloves, aprons, goggles and face masks commonly used. Gloves are indicated if I am to have any contact with wounds, bodily fluids or blood. Aprons are indicated if there is a risk of bodily fluids blood splashing onto my clothes. Goggles and face masks are indicated if there is a risk of splashing into my face or eyes.
- In many Trusts, patients who are isolated in a side room for infection control purposes also require healthcare professionals to wear an apron and gloves before entering the room.
- I am aware of other equipment such as respirators, which are used for airborne infections.

IMPORTANT INFECTION CONTROL ASPECTS TO CONSIDER WITH REGARD TO PPE

- All PPE should be stored in a clean and dry area to prevent contamination.
- If PPE has been damaged or contaminated, it should be discarded immediately.
- Due to the high risk of PPE becoming contaminated, it is essential that it is only worn for the shortest amount of time required during the procedure.

TYPES OF PPE

GLOVES AND APRONS

- Remember that gloves and aprons are to protect the healthcare worker and not the patient.
- Staff must not leave a single room or bay wearing gloves and/or aprons unless there is an emergency or there is potential risk of bodily fluid spillage; for example, when removing a bedpan.
- Gloves should never be decontaminated with alcohol gel or soap between use. They should also be changed immediately after each patient or completion of a procedure, even if on the same patient.
- Full-body gowns/fluid-repellent coveralls (instead of aprons) are indicated when there is extensive splashing of bodily fluids.
- These must be disposed of as clinical waste.

SURGICAL FACE MASKS

- Surgical face masks must be worn for surgery or when in contact with a patient who has a suspected/confirmed transmittable virus.
- They are a form of single-use PEE.
- They need to be secured tightly around the back of the head and at the nose bridge to ensure a good seal.
- They must be changed if contaminated or if they become wet.
- These must be disposed of as clinical waste.

FILTERING FACE PIECE (FFP) 3 DISPOSABLE RESPIRATOR MASKS

- FFP3 masks offer the highest level of respiratory protection. They filter particles that include viruses and bacteria.
- They are indicated when:
  - Undertaking aerosol-generating procedures on patients with confirmed or suspected respiratory pathogens.
  - Caring for patients with confirmed or suspected respiratory tuberculosis (TB), pandemic/avian influenza, Ebola or Middle East respiratory syndrome (MERS).

GOGGLES, VISORS AND FACE SHIELDS

- These are indicated when there is a risk of blood, body fluids, secretions and excretions splashing onto the face or into the eyes.
- Regular corrective glasses are not considered adequate eye protection. If indicated, goggles, a visor or face shield should be worn above the glasses.

DONNING AND DOFFING OF PPE

It is imperative that the donning (putting on) and doffing (removing) of PPE is performed in the correct sequence in order to minimise the risk of cross-infection and inadvertent contamination of the healthcare worker. Some general principles to bear in mind are:
- Put on PPE before entering the area where the patient is located.
- Keep your hands away from the face and PPE that is worn.
- Change gloves when they are torn or heavily contaminated.
- Limit the surfaces touched in patient environment.

Donning and doffing PPE is summarised for non-aerosol generating procedures in Figs 8.9 and 8.10, and for aerosol generating procedures in Figs 8.11 and 8.12.

Mark Scheme for Examiner

	0	1	2	3
Personal Protective Equipment				
Discusses indications				
Discusses common PPE, e.g. gloves, aprons				
Discusses less common PPE, e.g. respirators, goggles, visors, face shields				
Donning PPE				
Cleans hands				
Applies disposable single-use apron				
Applies face mask				
Ensures that face is not touched after face mask has been applied				
Applies eye protection if indicated				
Applies disposable non-sterile gloves				
Donning procedure done in the correct sequence				
Doffing PPE				
Correctly removes non-sterile gloves				
Immediately discards gloves into the clinical waste bin				
Cleans hands with alcohol gel				
Correctly removes disposable single-use apron,				
Immediately discards apron into the clinical waste bin				
Correctly removes eye protection				
Immediately discards it into the clinical waste bin				
Cleans hands with alcohol gel				
Ensures that all of the above steps are performed while still inside of the room or cohort area where patients are being cared for				
Once outside the room, correctly removes the face mask				
Immediately discards the face mask into the clinical waste bin				
Washes hands with soap and water				
Doffing procedure done in the correct sequence				

0 = Not attempted
1 = Performed, with room for improvement
2 = Adequately performed
3 = Performed beyond level expected

Pre-donning instructions:

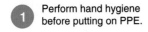
- Ensure healthcare worker hydrated
- Tie hair back

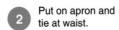
- Remove jewellery
- Check PPE in the correct size is available
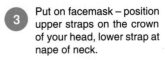

1 Perform hand hygiene before putting on PPE.

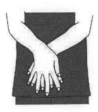

2 Put on apron and tie at waist.

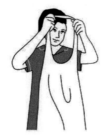
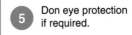

3 Put on facemask – position upper straps on the crown of your head, lower strap at nape of neck.

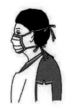

4 With both hands, mould the metal strap over the bridge of your nose.

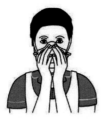

5 Don eye protection if required.

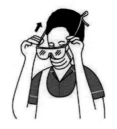

6 Put on gloves.

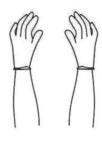

Fig. 8.9 Donning PPE for non–aerosol-generating procedures. (© Crown copyright)

❓ QUESTIONS AND ANSWERS FOR CANDIDATE

When should wearing a respirator (protective mask) be considered?
- Anyone coming in contact with a patient with a communicable disease spread through the air; for example, possible avian flu

Name five notifiable diseases within the UK.
- Acute encephalitis
- Acute infectious hepatitis
- Acute meningitis
- Acute poliomyelitis
- Anthrax
- COVID-19

What does the 'bare below the elbows' dress code mean, and when should it be followed?
- This dress code means that healthcare workers must avoid wearing jewellery, wrist bands, wrist watches and long sleeves and having long, false nails or nails with nail varnish on.
- This is followed by everyone when working in a clinical area or delivering direct patient care.

Name two occasions when you should use sterile gloves, and non-sterile gloves respectively.

Sterile gloves	Non-sterile gloves
• Any type of surgical procedure • Lumbar puncture • Urinary catheterisation • Suturing • Proctoscopy • Therapeutic paracentesis • Diagnostic or pleural ascitic tap • Chest drain • Knee joint aspiration	When in contact with blood, bodily fluids, microorganisms or chemicals. For example: • Cannulation • Venepuncture • Removal of peripheral cannula or urinary catheter • Taking a wound swab • Intravenous drug administration • Emptying or changing stoma bags, incontinence pads, commodes, bedpans, vomit bowls • Handling clinical waste or soiled linen • Nasogastric tube insertion • Setting up a giving set or blood transfusion

• **PPE should be removed in an order that minimises the risk of self-contamination**

• **Gloves, aprons (and eye protection if used) should be taken off in the patient's room or cohort area**

1 Remove gloves. Grasp the outside of glove with the opposite gloved hand; peel off.

Hold the removed glove in the remaining gloved hand.

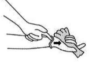

Slide the fingers of the un-gloved hand under the remaining glove at the wrist.

Peel the remaining glove off over the first glove and discard.

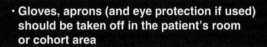

2 Clean hands.

3 Apron.

Unfasten or break apron ties at the neck and let the apron fold down on itself.

Break ties at waist and fold apron in on itself – do not touch the outside – **this will be contaminated.** Discard.

4 Remove eye protection if worn.

Use both hands to handle the straps by pulling away from face and discard.

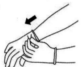

5 Clean hands.

6 Remove face mask once your clinical work is completed.

Untie or break bottom ties, followed by top ties or elastic, and remove by handling the ties only. Lean forward slightly. Discard. DO NOT reuse once removed.

7 Clean hands with soap and water.

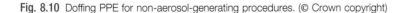

Fig. 8.10 Doffing PPE for non-aerosol-generating procedures. (© Crown copyright)

Use safe work practices to protect yourself and limit the spread of infection:

- Keep hands away from face and PPE being worn
- Change gloves when torn or heavily contaminated
- Limit surfaces touched in the patient environment
- Regularly perform hand hygiene
- Always clean hands after removing gloves

Pre-donning instructions

- ensure healthcare worker hydrated
- tie hair back
- remove jewellery
- check PPE in the correct size is available

Putting on personal protective equipment (PPE). The order for putting on is gown, respirator, eye protection and then gloves. This is undertaken outside the patient's room.

Perform hand hygiene before putting on PPE

1 **Put on the long-sleeved fluid repellent disposable gown** - fasten neck ties and waist ties.

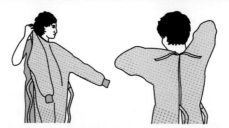

2 **Respirator-**

Note: This must be the respirator that you have been fit tested to use. Where goggles or safety spectacles are to be worn with the respirator, these must be worn during the fit test to ensure compatibility.

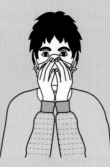

Position the upper straps on the crown of head, above the ears and the lower strap at the nape of the neck. Ensure that the respirator is flat against your cheeks. With both hands mould the nose piece from the bridge of the nose firmly, pressing down both sides of the nose with your fingers until you have fit. If a good fit cannot be achieved **DO**

Perform a fit check. The technique for this will differ between different makes of respirators. Instructions for the correct technique are provided by manufactures and should be followed for fit checking

3 **Eye protection** - place over face and eyes and adjust the headband to fit.

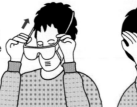

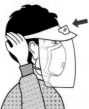

4 **Gloves** - select according to hand size. Ensure cuff of gown covered is covered by the cuff of the glove.

Fig. 8.11 Donning PPE for aerosol-generating procedures. (© Crown copyright)

PPE should be removed in an order that minimises the potential for cross contamination.

The order of removal of PPE is as follows:

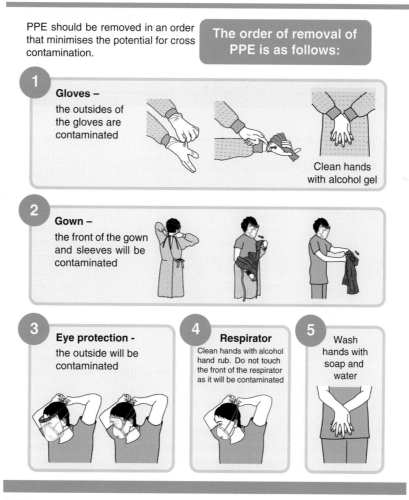

1 Gloves –
the outsides of the gloves are contaminated

Clean hands with alcohol gel

2 Gown –
the front of the gown and sleeves will be contaminated

3 Eye protection -
the outside will be contaminated

4 Respirator
Clean hands with alcohol hand rub. Do not touch the front of the respirator as it will be contaminated

5 Wash hands with soap and water

Fig. 8.12 Doffing PPE for aerosol-generating procedures. (© Crown copyright)

 Tip Box

Remember that face shields should always be used as an adjunct to other PPE, and not solely as protection from airborne pathogens, due to the lack of a good seal which could allow for aerosol penetration.

 Fact Box

Aerosol-generating procedures include: intubation or extubation, sputum induction, chest physiotherapy or suctioning, manual ventilation, tracheostomy, bronchoscopy, dental procedures, non-invasive ventilation, high-flow nasal oxygen.

GUIDELINES

WHO guidelines on hand hygiene in health care (No. WHO/ IER/PSP/2009/01). World Health Organization; 2009.

NICE, 2014. Infection prevention and control. Available at: www.nice.org.uk/guidance/qs61 (accessed 8 June 2022).

(2020) COVID-19 infection prevention and control guidance. https://www.gov.uk/government/publications/wuhan-novelcoronavirus-infection-prevention-and-control.

Index

Note: Page numbers followed by 'f' indicate figures those followed by 't' indicate tables and 'b' indicate boxes.